Present State and
Future Needs in
General Practice

Present State and Future Needs in General Practice

Sixth Edition

By

John Fry

Foreword by

John Lawson

President of the Royal College of General Practitioners

Published for

The Royal College of General Practitioners

by

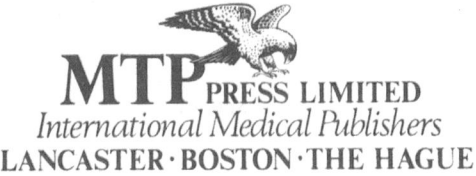

MTP PRESS LIMITED

International Medical Publishers

LANCASTER · BOSTON · THE HAGUE

Published in the United Kingdom and Europe
by MTP Press Limited
Falcon House, Lancaster, England

British Library Cataloguing in Publication Data

Present state and future needs in general practice—6th ed
1. Physicians (General practice)—Great Britain
I. Fry, John   II. Royal College of General Practitioners
   362.1'0425   R729.5.G4

Published in the USA
by MTP Press, A division of Kluwer Boston Inc.
190 Old Derby Street, Hingham, MA 02043, USA

Library of Congress Cataloging in Publication Data

Present state and future needs in general practice.
Includes index.
1. Family medicine—Great Britain. 2. Physicians
(General practice)—Great Britain. I. Fry, John,
1922-   II. Royal College of General Practitioners.
[DNLM: 1. Family practice—Trends—Great Britain.
W 89 P933]
R729.5.G4P73 1982   362.1   83-862

ISBN-13: 978-0-85200-708-2   e-ISBN-13: 978-94-011-7304-9
DOI: 10.1007/978-94-011-7304-9

Present State and Future Needs
  First Edition 1965
  Second Edition 1970
  Third Edition 1973
  Fourth Edition (Trends in General Practice 1977) 1977
  Fifth Edition (Trends in General Practice 1979) *1979*
  Sixth Edition (Present State and Future Needs in General Practice) *1983*

Typeset by Titus Wilson and Son Ltd., Kendal, England.

Bound by Pegasus Bookbinding, Melksham, Wiltshire.

Contents

Foreword

In the sixth edition of this work John Fry has reverted to the format of the earlier editions published in 1965, 1970 and 1973 and has presented statistical data drawn widely from many sources. General practice in the United Kingdom and elsewhere throughout the world has undergone many changes in the past decade. This new edition brings the available statistical information up to date and indicates the way ahead. General practice, the College and the National Health Service have been closely linked in effecting change. The membership of the College continues to grow and its influence in changing the face of general practice in the United Kingdom is significant.

John Fry's new book presents that characteristic blend of fact and personal opinion which was so successful in earlier editions and so valuable to general practice and others in primary health care. Once again he has shown what can be achieved by one man based on his own work and those of others in general practice.

RCGP, 1983

John Lawson
President of the Royal College
of General Practitioners

Preface

The *Present State and Future Needs* series had its roots in the dark days of the early 1960s when morale in general practice was low and when numbers of new entrants were actually going down. They were the days of mass emigration of doctors from Britain and the National Health Service.

The fourth and fifth editions were entitled *Trends in General Practice* (1977 and 1979).

Now, 20 years later, this sixth edition is produced in times of good morale for general practice and of serious crisis for the National Health Service.

As in previous editions, this one sets out to review data and facts on general practice in Britain. The information has come from a few sources. Most has been readily and willingly provided by the Department of Health and Social Security, the Scottish Home and Health Department and from Northern Ireland. The Office of Health Economics is another valuable source of information through its regular publications and its Compendia (the most recent published in 1981). The Councils of Postgraduate Education have provided facts on vocational training and continuing education. Intercontinental Medical Statistics through its continuing market research exercises can provide data on work patterns. The College has given details on its growing membership and examination.

To all these and many individuals I am grateful for their ready responses to my questions and requests.

However, the book is a personal work and inevitably the views expressed are my own and do not represent those of the College or any body with whom I am associated.

It is not intended to be a comprehensive study of all aspects of British general practice. Rather it demonstrates what data and facts are available, even if one has to dig them out. It does provide information on the structure and workings of general practice. It does not provide only consideration of the nature and process of clinical work.

More than anything else, it seeks to demonstrate what is possible in collecting and collating available data, but also to show what more needs to be done. Similar studies reviewing clinical, economic and behavioural aspects of general practice would be equally valuable.

Beckenham, Kent, 1983   John Fry

1
The place of general practice (primary health care)

General practice, the oldest form of medical care, has been redis-covered and renamed by medicopolitical administrators and planners. It is now *'primary health care'*, and it is recognized as so important that on it is based the hopes of 'Health Care for All: 2000' — the World Health Organization's (WHO) objective for the twenty-first century.

The World Health Organization's involvement in and concern for primary health care (PHC) has been demonstrated by pro-nouncements from its international meeting at Alma Ata in the USSR in 1978. Some quotations from Alma Ata are significant and helpful in setting the place and roles for primary health care, now and in the future.

* PHC is essential health care made universally accessible to individuals and families in the community by means acceptable to them, through their full participation and at a cost that the community and country can afford. It forms an integral part both of the country's health system, of which it is the nucleus, and of the overall social and economic development of the community.
* PHC addresses the main health problems in the community, providing promotive, preventive, curative and rehabilita-tive services accordingly.
* PHC is likely to be most effective if it employs means that are understood and accepted by the community and applied by community health workers (CHW) at a cost the com-

1

munity and the country can afford. The CHWs, including traditional practitioners where applicable, will function best if they reside in the community they serve and are trained socially and technically to respond to its expected health needs.
* Since PHC is an integral part both of the country's health system and of overall economic and social development, without which it is bound to fail, it has to be coordinated on a national basis with other levels of the health system as well as with the other sectors that contribute to a country's total development strategy.

These recommendations by the WHO to all the countries of the world are sound sensible principles that all should follow. They apply equally to the British National Health Service and they constitute such important recommendations that they merit restating.

* Primary health care being accessible and acceptable to the people is the essential basis and nucleus of every system of health care – it must be well integrated into the system.
* Primary health care has to be provided at a cost that the country can afford.
* Primary health care must be involved in care that is:
    * promotive
    * preventive
    * curative
    * rehabilitative
* Primary health care must be understood by the public through better health education and information.
* Those providing primary health care should include not only physicians but also other non-medical community health workers.

BRITISH GENERAL PRACTICE

The British National Health Service has always included general practice as an essential level of care.

Figure 1.1 depicts its place with the pyramid of care and its

2

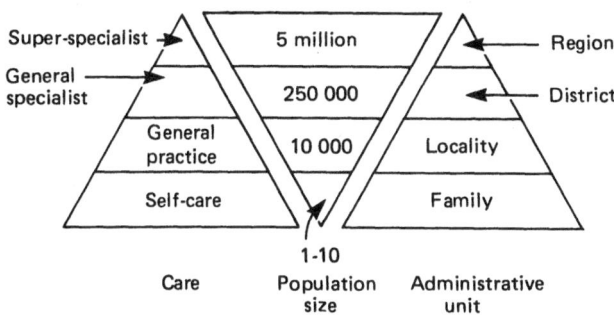

Figure 1.1   Levels of care

relationships to population size and administrative levels. It shows the *levels of care* in a health system.

Features of general practice

The main features of general practice are:

* available direct access to the practitioner in the community;
* portal of entry into the National Health Service; it is through the general practitioner that referral is made to the specialist services;
* first-contact care involving diagnosis and assessment of problems and needs;
* coordination and manipulation of medical and social services for the individual patient's and family's needs;
* relatively small and stable population base of 10 000 for a group of four general practitioners (or 2500 persons per general practitioner) (see Chapter 4);
* long-term and continuing personal care within the community by doctors of patients, well known to each other;
* the content of morbidity and mortality will be just that occurring in a population of 10 000 (or 2500) persons (see Chapter 3);
* care will be comprehensive including:
    * prevention of disease
    * promotion of health
    * cure of disease (when possible)
    * relief and comfort (when cure is not possible)

3

* rehabilitation of the disabled to ensure best use of individual functions and social resources.

Figure 1.2 shows some of the differences that exist between the primary health care level in the community and the general specialist services within a district general hospital.

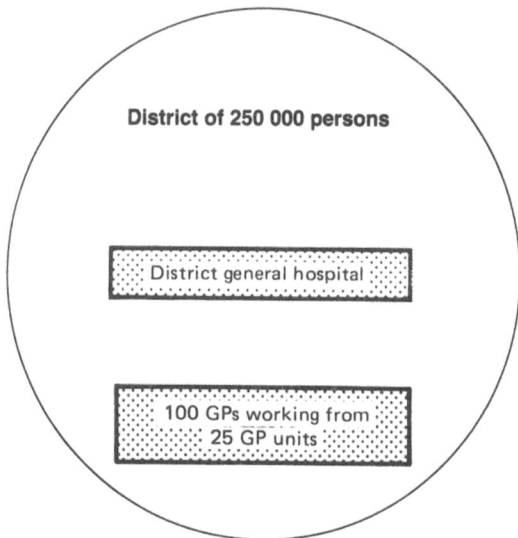

District of 250 000 persons

District general hospital

100 GPs working from 25 GP units

Figure 1.2   A district – with a district general hospital (DGH), GP units and individual GPs

Within a *district of 250 000 persons* there are likely to be:

* *a district general hospital* (one or a collection of smaller units);
* 25 *GP units* (group practices);
* 100 *GPs;*
* 250 000 *persons* involved in self-care.

Each level of care will care for most of its own particular problems without referral to the next level of care — but some referrals are necessary and expected.

* Thus more than three or four of all problems at the *self-care level* are managed without referral to a general practitioner or other primary health care service;

4

* Thus about eight episodes out of ten at the *general practitioner level* are managed without referral to the *district general hospital* (H).

Figure 1.3 depicts these proportions diagramatically.

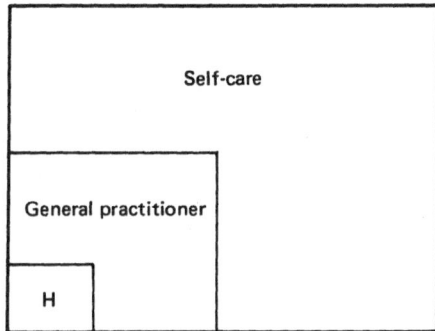

Figure 1.3   Proportions of care at levels of care

PRIMARY HEALTH CARE TEAM (PHC)

No longer is general practice carried out by single-handed practitioners working alone and in isolation (see Chapter 5).

Primary health care is now a 'team' exercise involving many community health workers. Doctors, nurses, receptionists, secretaries, social workers and others such as home-helps are all very much part of the team at the horizontal primary health care level (see Figure 1.1). The extent of the teamwork is variable (see Chapter 4).

Teamwork must also extend vertically to include cooperation and collaboration with the level of self-care and the public and with the general specialist services at the district level.

The concept of teamwork must include the WHO objectives of coordination of all services at local, district and national levels to achieve optimal quality from the available resources.

5

GENERAL PRACTICE — A SPECIAL FIELD

Primary health care, including general practice, is a special field of health care. It has its own:

* content of problems, and morbidity
* skills, tools, methods and techniques
* training, teaching and learning needs
* research needs.

It is a special field of care in all health systems with many basic international similarities common to all countries but also with differences of detail relating to the particular national system.

Therefore, there is much knowledge, experience, research data and educational methodology that can be shared and exchanged between countries.

2
What goes on?
A demography of general practice

POPULATION BASES

The basic unit of general practice is the *general practitioner* with an average practice population now of less than 2500 persons.

Whilst the individual general practitioner is still the key to long-term personal and family care, for demographic and planning purposes it is more appropriate to adopt the *group practice* as the basic unit. The mean number of general practitioners now is almost four (see Chapter 5).

Therefore, it is proposed that: *a group practice of four general practitioners caring for a population of 10 000 persons* be adopted as the demographic unit for primary health care. The four general practitioners are taken as 'whole time equivalents' (WTE), that is full time in *general practice*.

At present many general practitioners have outside professional commitments and are really 'part-timers'. So that there may be five or even six general practitioners in some practices caring for a practice population of 10 000 — nevertheless it is convenient to use the whole time equivalents of four general practitioners per 10 000.

POPULATION STRUCTURE

The age-distributions of populations of 10 000 and 2500 in the United Kingdom are shown in Table 2.1 and Figure 2.1.

Table 2.1   Age distributions of UK populations of 10 000 and 2500 (to nearest 10's and 100's)

Age	Numbers	
	per 10 000	per 2500
0–14	2500	620
15–44	4000	1000
45–64	2000	500
65–74	1000	250
75+	500	130
Total	10 000	2500

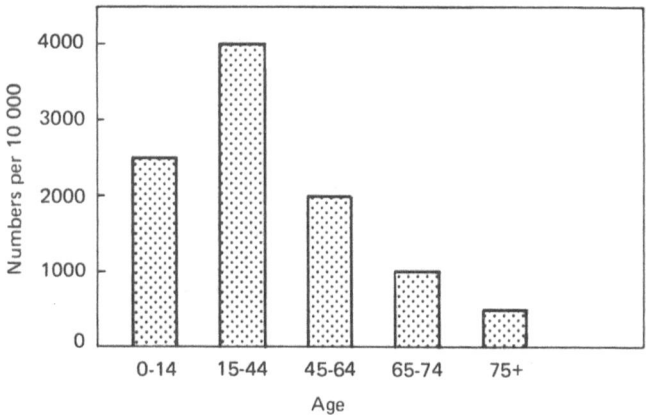

Figure 2.1   Age distribution of a UK population of 10 000

These population breakdowns show the numbers at risk in the various age-groups that have to be considered when plans are made for preventive and other community exercises.

For example, there are in a population of 10 000, 500 elderly persons aged over 75 years who are potentially vulnerable to social and medical crises and whom the practice nurses and health visitors may wish to visit or contact in a continuing preventive scheme.

ANNUAL BIRTHS

Tables 2.2 to 2.5 show the numbers of births and related events that may be expected in our basic populations.

Table 2.2   Annual births: numbers, infant mortality and primiparae

Annual events	Numbers per 10 000	per 2500
Total live births	128	32
Infant mortality including stillbirths	1–2	one every 4 years
Primiparae	42	11

Table 2.3   Annual births: place of delivery

Place of delivery – annual	Numbers per 10 000	per 2500
Hospital	126	32
GP hospital unit — if available	(60)	(15)
Home	2	less than 1

Table 2.4   Annual births: normal and abnormal

Annual events	Numbers per 10 000	per 2500	%
Normal deliveries	111	28	87
Forceps	13	3	10
Caesarean section	4	less than 1	3
Total	128	32	100

Table 2.5   Annual: abortions, terminations of pregnancy and women under family planning care

Annual events	Numbers per 10 000	per 2500
Spontaneous abortions	16	4
Termination of pregnancy	20	5
Family planning care	400	100

The numbers raise important issues in relation to decisions relating to the role of general practitioners in obstetrics.

* How many annual births are considered appropriate per general practitioner or per GP unit for continuing levels of experience and expertise?
* If normal deliveries (87% of all births) are to be the province of midwives (if not what should be their role?) and abnormal deliveries the responsibility of the specialist hospital obstetrics unit what is the role of the general practitioner in obstetric care?

Note: three forceps deliveries per 2500 population and less than one caesarean section per year. Even with 13 forceps deliveries per year in a GP unit of 10 000 persons it is likely that many of these will be carried out by the specialist hospital service.

Whatever the distribution of roles and duties between general practice, hospitals and other local agencies (such as family planning clinics) the large numbers of women involved make the case for effective and safe maternity–obstetric services very obvious.

The distribution and sharing of care between general practitioners, community midwives, health visitors and hospital obstetric services need to be planned, organized, administered and audited regularly in each district in a cooperative and collaborative manner to ensure optimal care and results.

ANNUAL DEATHS

Just over one-quarter of deaths now take place at home (Table 2.6). Two-thirds take place in hospitals, and this proportion is

Table 2.6   Annual deaths: place of death

Annual deaths – place	Numbers		%
	per 10 000	per 2500	
Home	30	7	27
Hospital	70	18	64
Elsewhere	10	3	9
Total	110	28	100

increasing. The 'elsewhere' category includes sudden deaths in public places and in the street and in nursing homes and hospices. In spite of the publicity deaths in hospices account for only about 2% of deaths in the United Kingdom.

Causes of death

The causes of death are shown in Table 2.7. The numbers are appreciable of families affected by grief and bereavement,

Table 2.7   Annual deaths: causes

Annual deaths	Numbers per 10 000	per 2500
Heart diseases	40	10
Cancers	20	5
Respiratory diseases	20	5
Strokes	15	4
Accidents (violent)	8	2
Suicide	1	(one every 4 years)
Others	6	2
Total	110	28

spouses in widowhood (or widowers), and families in the terminal care process, whether the deaths are in hospital or at home – 110 in a group practice – representing considerable family care and support.

The main causes of death are heart diseases, cancers, respiratory diseases, and strokes.

Terminal care at home involving nursing and doctor support probably involves some 20 deaths in the group practice or five for the individual general practitioner.

Of the 20, eight will be deaths from chronic heart failure, seven from cancers, five from chronic respiratory disease and five from strokes.

GENERAL PRACTITIONER ACTIVITIES IN VARIOUS SERVICES

The average NHS general practitioner now is a *part-timer*. Up to 40% of his professional time may be spent working in hospitals, in schools or homes for aged and handicapped, in clinics, on boards or commissions, on insurance work, or in teaching and training. Also there are some practitioners such as married women or elderly doctors who are part-timers by choice.

It should be noted that *private practice* outside the NHS is a very small part of general practice in the United Kingdom – probably less than 5% of total volume of work.

6·4% of the population (3·6 million) are covered by private health schemes for specialist and hospital services.

Certain of the general practitioner's activities are definable, apart from the traditional consultations and home visits. Tables 2.8 and 2.9 provide a composite collection of possible numbers involved in preventive tasks – of course much preventive care is carried out in the context of the consultation.

Table 2.8   Annual GP services: obstetrics and gynaecology

Annual numbers of persons (possible)	Numbers	
	per 10 000	per 2500
Family planning	400	100
Antenatal clinic (weekly attendances)	35	9
Termination of pregnancy	20	5
Cervical cytology	400 (two to three positive smears)	100 (one positive smear every 2 years)

Table 2.9   Annual GP services: child welfare and immunization

Annual numbers of persons (possible)	Numbers	
	per 10 000	per 2500
Child welfare clinics		
New babies (0–1 year)	15–20 per week	4–5 per week
Children (1–5 years)	10–15 per week	2–3 per week
Immunizations		
Children	22 per week	5 per week
Adults	3 per week	1 per week

Table 2.8 shows the large numbers of services involved in

preventive work in the obstetrics and gynaecology field, and Table 2.9 the large numbers involved in child care and immunizations. Taken together the numbers show the need for good organization of such work.

3
Content of work

General practice provides a broad clinical spectrum of true morbidity in the community. Hospital practice is involved mainly with only that small proportion of morbidity referred there by general practitioners. Figure 3.1 shows that whilst some disorders are self-managed the general practitioner is involved with the great majority of serious morbidity. Even those cases which may be managed for some time in hospital will come from general practice where the initial assessment and diagnosis have to be made, and which return to general practice for aftercare.

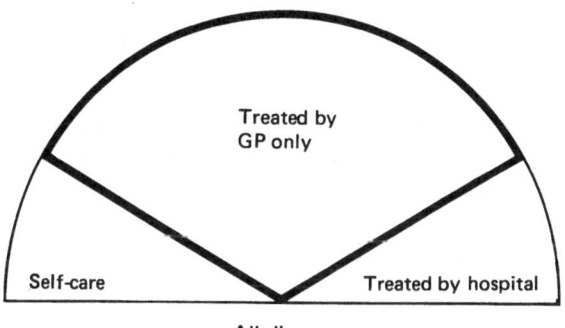

Figure 3.1   Spectrum of care

SEVERITY OF DISEASE

General practice is the level of first-contact. It is the level of care to which the public bring their undefined and unselected

15

packages of health problems that have to be assessed and diagnosed by the general practitioner.

Hospital practice deals with more selected and defined clinical material largely categorized and referred to it by local practitioners.

Since 'common diseases commonly occur and rare diseases rarely happen' it is inevitable that general practice (primary health care) will be involved with common conditions, which tend to be relatively minor and self-limiting and with chronic disorders that tend to be long-lasting and non-curable. Dramatic life-threatening acute major situations are uncommon in general practice, though common at the district general hospital level.

Table 3.1 shows the proportions of these three grades of severity of disease in general practice.

Table 3.1 Disease in general practice: grades of severity

Severity	Per cent of patients consulting
Minor – self-limiting	65
Chronic – long-lasting and non-curable	25
Acute major – life-threatening	10
	100

CLINICAL CONTENT

Tables 3.2 and 3.3 are estimates of likely annual numbers of persons consulting in a group practice of 10 000 or seen by a general practitioner with 2500 patients.

General minor conditions

The general minor conditions that occur in general practice are, in order of frequency:

* upper respiratory infections
* skin disorders
* psychoemotional problems
* minor accidents
* gastrointestinal
* rheumatic aches and pains.

16

Table 3.2 General minor conditions in general practice: annual person consulting rates

Condition	Annual persons consulting	
	per 10 000	per 2500
Upper respiratory infections	2400	600
Skin disorders	1400	350
Psychoemotional problems	1000	250
Minor accidents	1000	250
Gastrointestinal conditions	800	200
Rheumatic aches and pains	600	150
'Symptoms'	1500	375

Table 3.3 Specific minor conditions in general practice: annual person consulting rates

Condition	Annual persons consulting	
	per 10 000	per 2500
Acute throat infections	400	100
Lacerations	400	100
Eczema–dermatitis	400	100
Acute otitis media	300	75
Ear wax	200	50
Urinary tract infections	200	50
Acute backache	200	50
Vaginal discharge	120	30
Migraine	100	25
Hay fever	100	25
Vertigo	80	20
Hernia	60	15
Piles	60	15

These are presented under such broad general diagnostic labels because in many no reliable specific diagnosis is possible. They do emphasize, however, what clinical groups are most prevalent in the community.

In addition there are those problems whose diagnosis can go no further than the presenting 'symptom'.

Such then is the true clinical content of general practice.

Table 3.3 goes a step further and gives estimates of persons consulting annually with *minor conditions to which more specific diagnoses can be attached.*

17

Note that the most prevalent seven diagnoses are:

* acute throat infections
* lacerations
* eczema–dermatitis
* acute otitis media
* ear wax
* urinary tract infections.
* acute backache

Chronic diseases

Chronic diseases (Table 3.4) in general practice feature more prominently than the dramatic acute major situations and minor

Table 3.4 Chronic diseases in general practice: annual person consulting rate

Conditions	Annual persons consulting	
	per 10 000	per 2500
High blood pressure	1000	250
Chronic rheumatism	400	100
(osteoarthroses)	(300)	(75)
(rheumatoid arthritis)	(40)	(10)
Chronic psychiatric	400	100
Ischaemic heart disease	200	50
Obesity	200	50
Congestive cardiac failure	160	40
Anaemia	120	30
(pernicious anaemia)	(20)	(5)
Cancers under care	120	30
Asthma	120	30
Diabetes	120	30
Varicose veins	120	30
Peptic ulcers	100	25
Strokes	80	20
Thyroid disorders	40	10
Epilepsy	40	10
Multiple sclerosis	12	3
Parkinsonism	12	3
Chronic renal failure	2	less than 1

conditions – because they are long-lasting and non-curable they require much time, support and resources over many years.

18

Note that the following five conditions are the most frequent:

* high blood pressure
* chronic rheumatism
* chronic psychiatric problems
* ischaemic heart disease
* obesity

Note also the numbers of persons consulting annually for disorders that require special supervision and control:

* high blood pressure
* anemia
* diabetes
* thyroid diseases
* epilepsy.

Major diseases

Life-threatening major diseases may be numerically few, but are important for early diagnosis, definitive treatment and after-care.

The most prevalent are the following six:

* acute chest infections
* severe depression
* acute myocardial infarction
* strokes
* cancers
* acute appendicitis.

Table 3.5 provides perspectives of the approximate numbers that may be expected annually.

It is helpful to break cancers down into the various sites as shown in Table 3.6. This shows the rarity of most cancers in a practice of 2500 persons.

Table 3.5   Major diseases in general practice: annual person consulting rates

Condition	Annual persons consulting	
	per 10 000	per 2500
Acute bronchitis	400	100
Pneumonia	80	20
Severe depression	40	10
(parasuicide)	(16)	(4)
(suicide)	(1)	(1 every 4 years)
Acute myocardial infarction	40	10
(sudden death)	(20)	(5)
Acute strokes	20	5
All new cancers	20	5
Acute appendicitis	15	4

Table 3.6   New cancers in general practice: annual patient consulting rates

Condition: new cancer	Annual persons consulting	
	per 10 000	per 2500
All new cancers	20	5
Lung	8	2
Breast	4	1
Large gut	3	2 in 3 years
Stomach	2	1 in 2 years
Prostate	2	1 in 2 years
Bladder	1	1 in 3 years
Cervix	1	1 in 4 years
Ovary	3 in 4 years	1 in 5 years
Oesophagus	1 in 2 years	1 in 7 years
Brain	1 in 3 years	1 in 10 years
Lymphadenoma	1 in 4 years	1 in 15 years
Thyroid	1 in 5 years	1 in 20 years

Social pathology

Social pathology is as prevalent as clinical pathology and as important. Working in the community the general practitioner naturally becomes involved in the social problems that exist. Table 3.7 gives the estimated prevalence of social problems. Their effects on individuals and families can only be imagined.

Congenital conditions

These are rare, but how rare is shown in Table 3.8.

Table 3.7 Social pathology in general practice

Condition	Annual prevalence	
	per 10 000	per 2500
'Poverty' and handicap		
Supplementary benefits		
elderly	240	60
non-elderly	240	60
attendance allowance	480	120
mobility allowance	320	80
invalidity allowance	1000	250
unemployed	400	100
Marriage, divorce, etc.		
marriages	48	12
divorces	16	4
one-parent families	160	40
Crime etc.		
burglaries	100	25
in prison	16	4
drunken driving	20	5
sexual assaults	4	1
juvenile delinquents	40	10
children in care	12	3

Table 3.8 Congenital abnormalities: incidence

Congenital Abnormality	Incidence	
	per 10 000	per 2500
Cardiac	2 every 3 years	1 every 5 years
Pyloric stenosis	1 every 2 years	1 every 7 years
Spina bifida	1 every 2 years	1 every 8 years
Down's syndrome	1 every 3 years	1 every 10 years
Cleft palate	1 every 5 years	1 every 20 years
Congenital dislocation of hip	1 every 5 years	1 every 20 years
Phenylketonuria	1 every 50 years	1 every 200 years

4
The primary health care team

Since the NHS began in 1948 there has been a steady trend away from the single-handed do-it-all-himself general practitioner towards the primary health care team.

To begin with, there was the steady build-up of partnership practice, but it has only been since the mid-1960s the concept of the primary health care team has grown.

In 1965–66 the General Practice Charter produced by the then Minister of Health, the British Medical Association and the Royal College of General Practitioners resulted in financial inducements for group practice of three or more partners and reimbursement (70%) of salaries of staff employed by general practitioners. In addition attachment of local authority employed district nurses, health visitors and community midwives was encouraged.

THE NUCLEUS PRACTICE UNIT

The mean number of general practitioners per practice or GP unit now is almost four – it was less than two in the 1960s.

Table 4.1 shows a typical nucleus practice unit and the members of the team.

It should be realized that in addition to general practice there are other direct-access primary services in the social-health field such as social workers, family planning services, child welfare, voluntary services, opticians, pharmacists, and various fringe medicine practitioners. Their relationships with general practice must be clarified in the future.

Table 4.1   Members of nucleus primary health care team per 10 000 population

Worker	Numbers
General practitioners	4
Practice manager	1
Medical secretaries/ receptionists	6–7 whole time equivalents (= 12 part timers)
Nurse (practice-employed)	1 in 3 practice units
Nurse (attached district nurses)	2–3
Health visitors	1–2
Midwife	1 per 3 practices

Numbers

The estimated numbers of primary health care workers in the United Kingdom are shown in Table 4.2.

Table 4.2   Primary health care workers in the United Kingdom (estimated numbers 1980)

Workers	Estimated numbers in United Kingdom in 1980 (whole time equivalents)
General practitioners	29 240
District nurses	20 000
Practice-employed nurses	3500
Health visitors	9000
Community midwives	3500
Practice-employed secretaries/receptionists	45 000
Social workers	24 300
Home helps	50 000

5
General practitioners: numbers

The numbers of general practitioners in the NHS should be related to other health workers.

MEDICAL AND NURSING MANPOWER
Over 1.5 million are employed in the NHS. Table 5.1 shows the numbers in 1981 of doctors and nurses employed in the NHS: they total over half a million.

Table 5.1   NHS medical and nursing staff (1981 estimated)

Country	Doctors and dentists in hospitals	Doctors in community medicine	Nurses and midwives	General practitioners
England	33 900	4300	370 100	23 740
Wales	2000	300	24 400	1500
Scotland	5300	800	58 600	3300
Northern Ireland	1500	200	17 300	800
Totals	42 700	5600	470 400	29 240

In addition to the 77 540 doctors in the NHS in 1981 there were estimated to be a further 3500 doctors working clinically in the United Kingdom outside the NHS – thus 95.5 per cent of all doctors in the United Kingdom are employed by the NHS.

NUMBERS OF GENERAL PRACTITIONERS
The numbers of general practitioners have been increasing since the mid-1960s. Table 5.2 shows the numbers from 1950 to 1981. There was an actual fall between 1960 and 1965 when general practice was in a depressed state but in other time periods a

progressive rise has occurred. Note the decline in numbers of
'assistants' and the rise in 'trainees' (Figures 5.1 and 5.2)

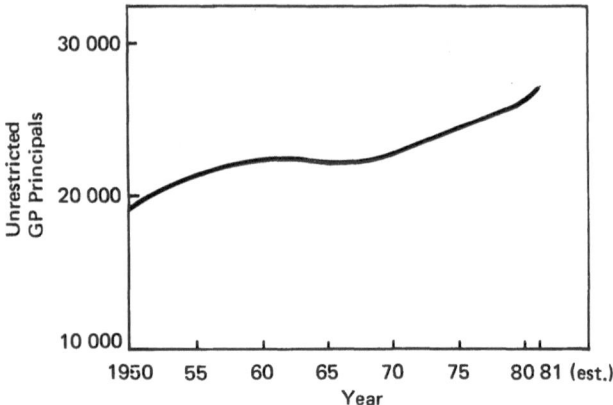

Figure 5.1   General practitioners in the NHS – 1950–81

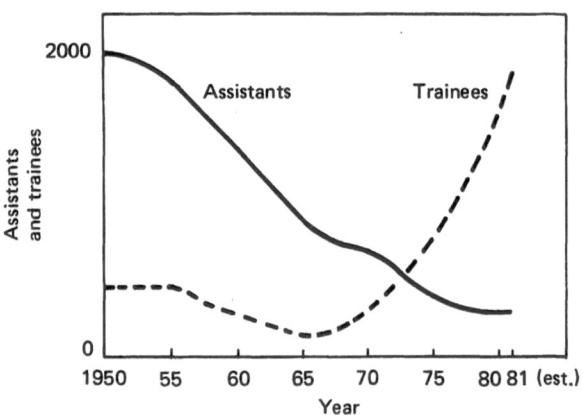

Figure 5.2   Numbers of trainees and assistants

Table 5.2   General practitioners in the NHS: 1950-81

Numbers	1950	1955	1960	1965	1970	1975	1980	1981 (estim.)
Unrestricted GP principals	19 000	21 150	22 620	22 400	22 961	24 644	26 143	27 100
Assistants	2000	1800	1335	820	727	441	305	300
Trainees	450	450	257	154	273	882	1704	1840
Totals	21 450	23 400	24 212	23 374	23 951	25 967	28 152	29 240

PERSONS PER GENERAL PRACTITIONER

In 1950 the mean numbers of persons per general practitioner (average list size) was 2500. By 1981 it had gone down to 1915 and it was likely to continue to go down because of increasing numbers of general practitioners in a relatively static population (Table 5.3, Figure 5.3).

Table 5.3   Persons per GP 1950-81 (UK)

	1950	1955	1960	1965	1970	1975	1980	1981
Persons per general practitioner	2500	2300	2257	2407	2413	2307	2017	1915

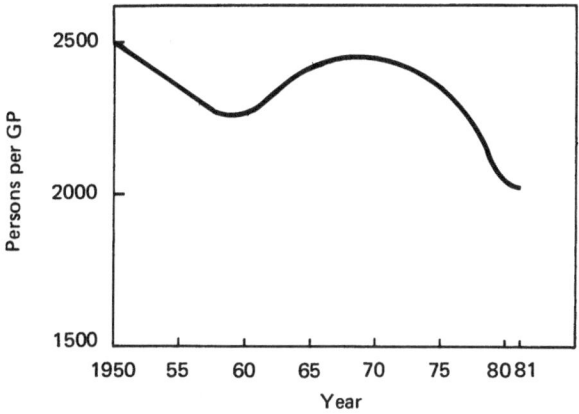

Figure 5.3   Persons per GP – 1950–81

Figure 5.4 shows that the average list rose in England and Wales, Scotland and Northern Ireland in 1951 and declined in 1980 in England and Wales and Scotland, but rose in Northern Ireland (as a result of emigration from the latter area).

27

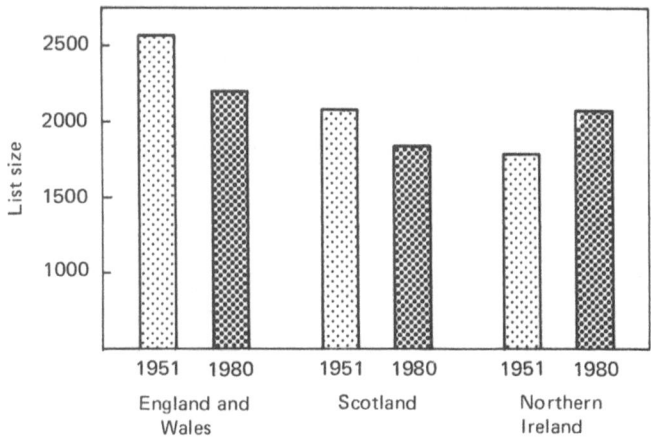

Figure 5.4   Changes in average list sizes per general practitioner in England and Wales, Scotland and Northern Ireland – 1951 and 1980

6
General practitioner profile

The average British general practitioner is male, in his early 40s, trained both in a provincial medical school and as a vocational trainee.

AGE

Table 6.1 and Figure 6.1 show the age distribution of general practitioners in the NHS.

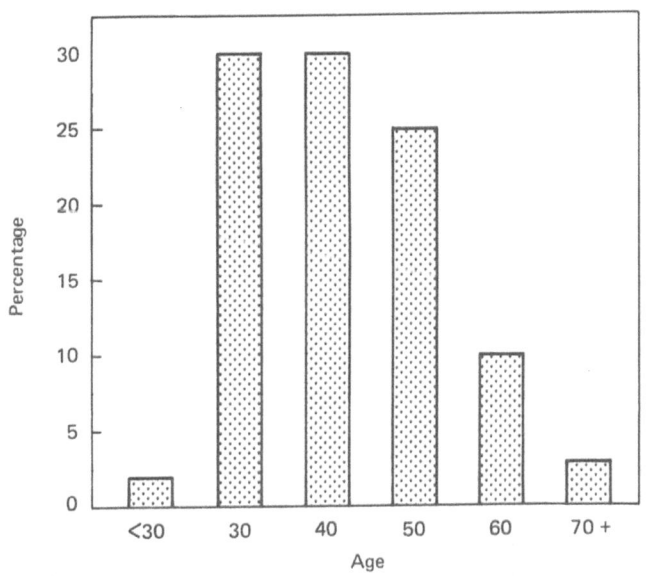

Figure 6.1   NHS general practitioners: age distribution

Table 6.1   NHS general practitioners: age distribution

Age	<30	30	40	50	60	70+	
%	2	30	30	25	10	3	100

SEX

Although the proportion of women general practitioners is increasing they still make up less than 20% of the general practitioner population (Table 6.2, Figure 6.2).

Table 6.2   NHS general practitioners: percentage of males and females

%	1970	1980
Male	90	83
Female	10	17
	100	100

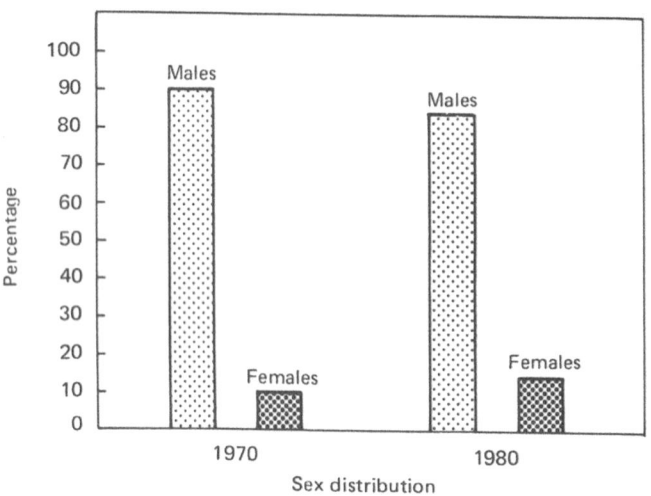

Figure 6.2   NHS general practitioners: percentage of males and females

PLACE OF GRADUATION

The proportion of foreign medical graduates (FMGs), that is NHS general practitioners born and graduated in other countries has risen to 19% of all general practitioners (Table 6.3, Figure 6.3). The number from Eire has declined.

Table 6.3   NHS general practitioners: place of birth and graduation

	Place of birth and graduation			
	Great Britain	Eire and Channel Islands	Elsewhere	
1970	77	9	14	100
1980	76	5	19	100

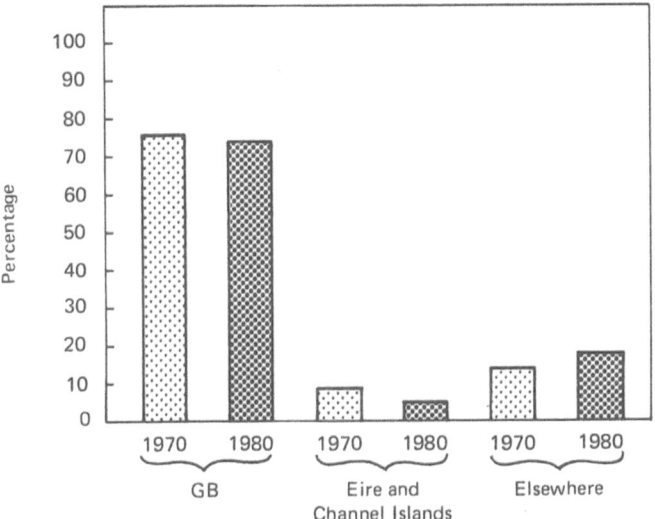

Figure 6.3   NHS general practitioners: place of birth and graduation

31

7
Practice units

The trend towards group practice continues but it is not towards very large groups.

The number of health centres being opened, built or planned is now much lower than in the expansionist period of the 1970s.

PRACTICE UNITS

The changes in sizes of general practice units from 1952 to 1980 are shown in Table 7.1 and Figure 7.1.

Table 7.1   Proportional distribution of NHS principals in England and Wales by size of practice

Size of practice unit (number of general practitioners)	1952 (17 204 unrestricted principals)	1980 (23 184 unrestricted principals)
1	43%	14%
2	33%	18%
3	15%	24%
4	6%	20%
5	2%	12%
over 6	1%	12%
	100%	100%
Mean	1.3	3.7

Single-handed practitioners in 1952 made up nearly one-half (43%) of the total, whereas by 1980 they only formed 14%. However, there are also very large group practices in Britain, but those with six or more partners form only 12% of the total.

33

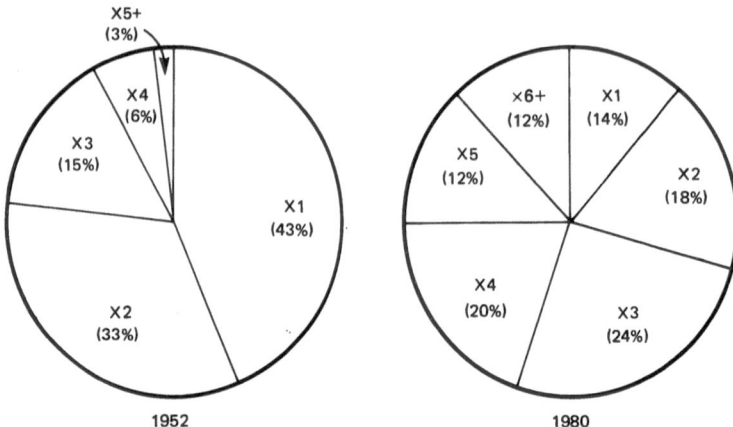

Figure 7.1   Proportions of general practice units

Taking the averages of the two years 1952 and 1980 – in 1952 the average practice was 1.3 practitioners and in 1980 it was 3.7.

The typical British general practice unit now consists of three to four general practitioners working as a group and caring for 6000-10 000 persons. Such a unit provides a compromise between the small and the large unit, and also between centralization of community health resources and accessibility for the local population.

HEALTH CENTRES

In the United Kingdom, by 1980 one-quarter of all general practitioners were providing and one-quarter of the population were using health centres.

The health centre expansion occurred chiefly in the 1970s following the general practitioner charter of 1965–6 which encouraged their building and offered inducements to practitioners to work in them. However, with changes in national health policies since 1979 the health centre movement has been drastically reduced.

The numbers of health centres in the United Kingdom, and the numbers of general practitioners working in them, are shown in Table 7.2.

Table 7.2   NHS 1980 health centres (numbers), numbers of general practitioners
working from them and percentages of all general practitioners

	Health centres	General practitioners	Per cent of all general practitioners
England	953	5189	24%
Wales	90	342	23%
Scotland	137	521	16%
Northern Ireland	70	446	58%
United Kingdom	1250	6498	24%

LONDON AND THE REST

The problems of the large inner cities continue a major concern, and those problems related to general practice are but one aspect.

Brian Jarman in *A Survey of Primary Care in London* (Occasional Paper 16, Royal College of General Practitioners, 1981) shows some of the differences between London and England and Wales, relating to both general practice services and social problems. Figures 7.2 (*a*) to (*e*) and 7.3 (*a*) to (*h*) show some of these differences in graphic form.

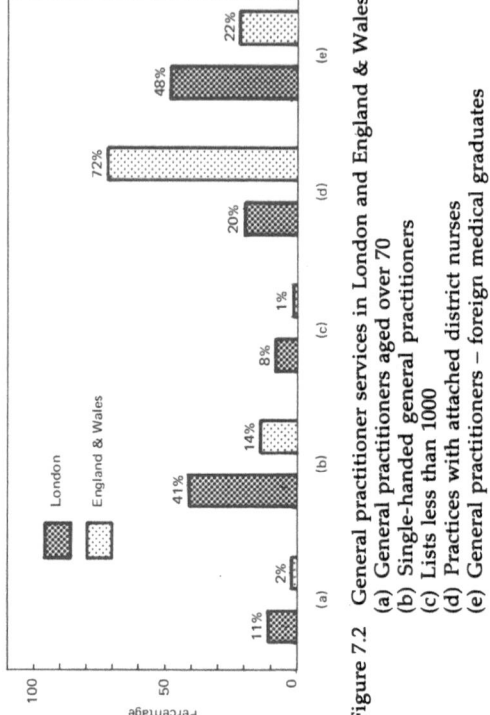

Figure 7.2   General practitioner services in London and England & Wales
(a) General practitioners aged over 70
(b) Single-handed general practitioners
(c) Lists less than 1000
(d) Practices with attached district nurses
(e) General practitioners – foreign medical graduates

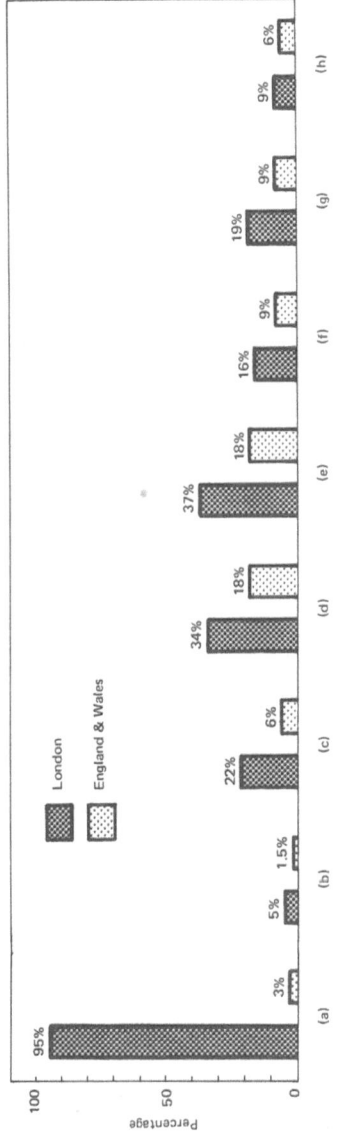

Figure 7.3 Social problems in London and England & Wales
(a) Population density: persons per hectare
(b) Overcrowding
(c) Foreigners
(d) One-person households
(e) Householders lacking amenities
(f) One-parent families
(g) Illegitimate births (% of all births)
(h) Mobility (% moving house per year)

8
Education and training

General practice is recognized as a special field of medicine with its own education and training requirements. The past 15 years have seen remarkable changes in education and training for general practice.

UNDERGRADUATE EDUCATION

The recommendations of the General Medical Council have been heeded by all medical schools. In all of the 28 medical schools there are periods of attachment to a general practice. All medical schools apart from Bristol have departments of general practice.

The strength and involvement of the departments of general practice varies from school to school. It appears that at Cambridge University, Charing Cross Hospital, King's College Hospital and Oxford University Medical Schools the representation and recognition of general practice departments is less than at the other 23 medical schools (Bristol has no department at all).

VOCATIONAL TRAINING

Since 1982 a 3-year approved training for general practice principals has become mandatory.

Vocational training for general practice has become a very large process – about one practice in four is recognized for vocational training. There are more general practice trainees than trainees for any other specialty.

Table 8.1 and Figure 8.1 show the numbers of practices,

trainers and trainees in 1981. One in four practices is involved in training and one in ten of all principals is a recognized trainer. In some practices there are more than one trainer. The numbers of trainers have always exceeded those of trainees.

Table 8.1   Numbers of teaching practices, trainers and trainees in 1981

	England and Wales	Scotland	Northern Ireland	Total	% of all
Training practices	1810	250	67	2127	24
Trainers	2234	306	88	2628	9
Trainees	1703	298	44	2045	

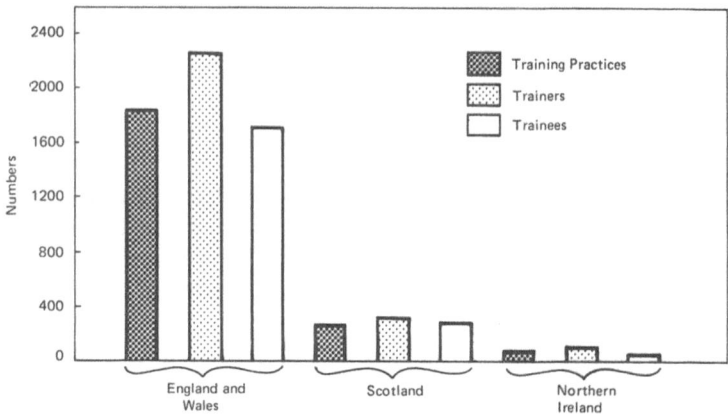

Figure 8.1   Numbers of teaching practices, trainers and trainees (1981)

Table 8.2 and Figure 8.2 show the rapid increase in trainers and trainees. From 1971 to 1981 the numbers of trainers quadrupled and the numbers of trainees increased 7-fold.

Table 8.2   Numbers of general practitioner trainers and trainees in the United Kingdom in 1971 and 1981

	1971 (Estimated)	1981
Trainers	650	2628
Trainees	300	2045

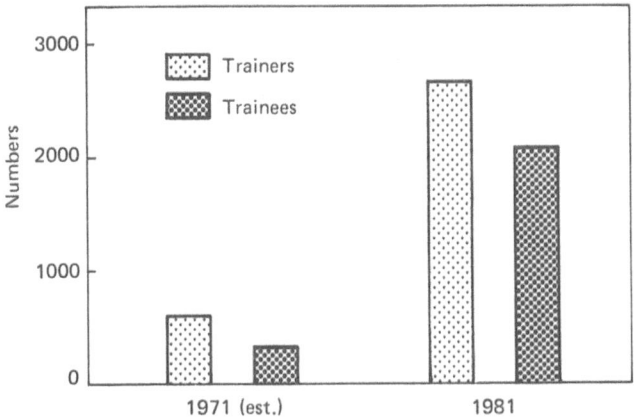

Figure 8.2   Numbers of general practitioners and trainees in the UK in 1971 and 1981

There are 250 vocational training courses. The average numbers of trainees per year is between four and six, so a course will have twelve to eighteen over the 3-year programme.

TRAINEES AND THE MRCGP EXAMINATION

In 1979–80 there were 1046 candidates for the MRCGP examination, of whom 480 were trainees. In 1982–3 there were over 1200 candidates.

It is not possible to relate present numbers of trainees (2045) with numbers of trainees taking the MRCGP exam (480)· in 1979–80. However, it is likely that in future the majority of trainees will take the MRCGP.

CONTINUING MEDICAL EDUCATION

There are 430 postgraduate medical centres based at NHS hospitals. All are involved in offering continuing medical education for general practitioners and others.

However, between 1975 and 1980 the attendances by general practitioners (recognized under Section 63) at these postgraduate medical centres fell by over one-quarter from 200 000 sessions in 1975 to 172 000 in 1980.

There may be various reasons for this fall in attendances, one of which being that general practitioners in the NHS no longer need to attend for a minimum number of sessions to be eligible to receive seniority awards.

9
Volume of work

The essence of general practice is its individuality. Each practitioner creates his own personal style of work related to his personality and medical philosophy. This applies not only to his clinical approach but also to the organization of his practice work.

Attempts to measure, record and analyse the volume of work in general practice are made difficult by the absence of reliable detailed information.

Most of the data comes from reports of the General Household Surveys (GHS) that rely on interviews with randomized samples of the population, on the Royal College of General Practitioners surveys (NMS) carried out in 1955–56 and 1970–71 (the third one was carried out in 1982), on results from data recorded by general practitioners for market research organizations such as IMS (Intercontinental Medical Statistics Ltd.), and on published papers by individual general practitioners.

The published mass surveys of GHS, NMS and IMS produce 'mass' averages. However, they do not demonstrate one of the special features of medical practice – the differences between individual practices and practitioners.

In the second NMS there were almost 150 general practitioners taking part. Their work-volume as measured by consultations per population at risk differed among these individual practitioners by almost 4-fold.

In addition to the influence of the practitioner's personality and philosophy, and these are the most potent factors that influence work-volume, there are others such as the health and morbidity, and social and medical expectations of the district, and

43

local back-up facilities in hospital and community services. The policies of the practice itself will also influence the organization and distribution of work.

In spite of all these provisos it is nevertheless useful to consider the available facts.

PATIENTS CONSULTING

In any and every year between 60 and 70% of the population consult their general practitioners at least once and some many times. Over 5 years about 90% of patients registered will consult their general practitioners.

PATIENT CONSULTATION NOTES

In the British NHS the public register with a general practitioner and he/she is paid an annual capitation fee for all persons registered. The population per general practitioner is a definite figure that serves as the denominator for calculating rates.

Provided that the numbers of consultations (or other services) are recorded it is possible to calculate the patient consultation rates over a period of time. Such consultation rates serve as a useful measure of work in general practice.

It is these patient consultation rates that vary so much among general practitioners. In the second NMS they ranged from a high of 6.6 annual consultations per person to a low of 1.8. Consultation rates vary with the age of the patients and Figure 9.1 shows this with highest rates in the young and the elderly.

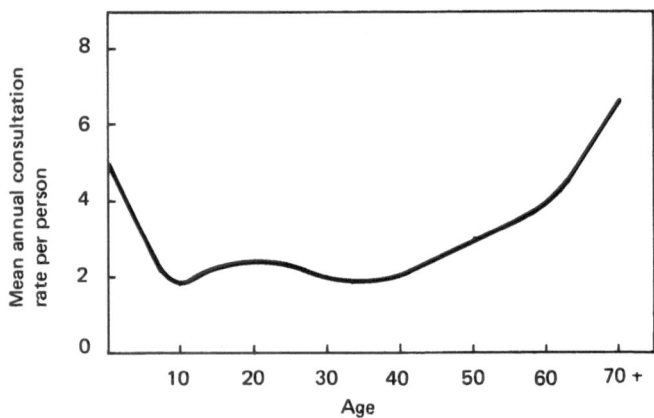

Figure 9.1   Mean annual consultation rates by age group (males: 3·55; females: 4·5)

The *annual patient consultation rates* reported have been as follows:

* NMS (1) (1955–56): 3.74
* NMS (2) (1970–71) 3.01
* GHS   (1971): 3.8
* GHS   (1977): 3.7

In all reports the annual consultation rates for females have been greater than for males by a figure of approximately one consultation; that is, for the NMS (2) mean rate of 3.01, that for females was 3.6 and for males 2.5.

To show that the consultation rates are not static in any practice, Figure 9.2 shows the annual rates in the author's own practice from 1950 to 1981.

The points to note are the higher rates in 1950–65 (3.5–4.0) followed by a fall and then a constant rate around 2.0 since 1970.

Most of the fall has been the result of a decline in the numbers of home visits; there has also been a decline in surgery consultation, but a marked increase in repeat prescriptions and in sharing work with a nurse and a health visitor.

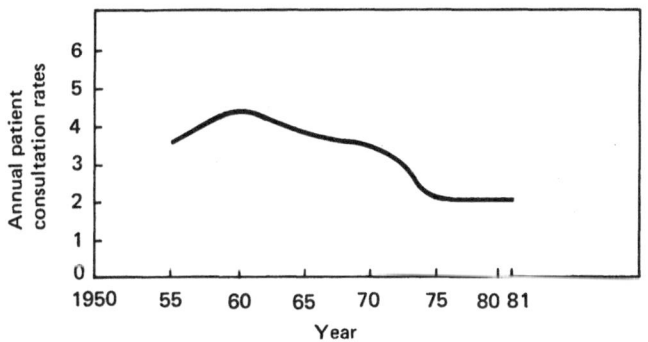

Figure 9.2   Annual patient consultation rates in a practice 1950–81

NIGHT VISITING

The average general practitioner may expect a night visit about once every 2 weeks. The numbers more than doubled from 1967 to 1976 (Table 9.1).

Table 9.1 Annual night visits per GP principal (1967–76) (from M. J. Buxton, R. F. Klein and J. Sayers, *British Medical Journal* (1977), 1, 827–30)

	Annual night visiting rates based on NHS claims per general practitioner principal
1967	11
1971	14
1976	24

The highest rates were in Tynemouth, Salford and Manchester with 40 annual night visits per general practitioner and the lowest were in Bath, Ipswich, Chester and Northampton with ten annual night visits. Highest rates were associated with availability of deputizing services and high proportion of social class V in the population.

OTHER WORK BOTH INSIDE AND OUTSIDE THE PRACTICE

Face-to-face consultations are but a part of the general practitioner's work.

A study by the RCGP Research Unit at Birmingham (1982) showed that apportioning time and services the approximate distribution of work in general practice was as shown in Table 9.2 and Figure 9.3.

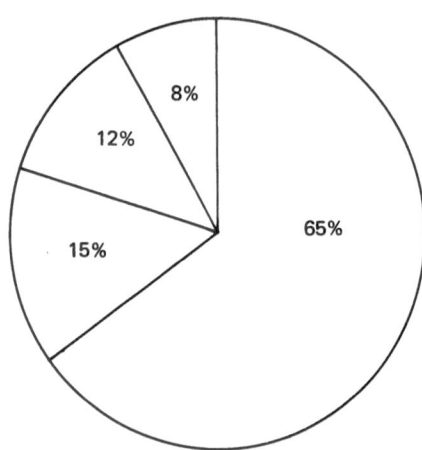

Figure 9.3 General practitioners' work load from Birmingham Research Unit, *Journal of the Royal College of General Practitioners* (1982), 32, 292–7

Table 9.2   General practitioners' work load (from Birmingham Research Unit, *Journal of the Royal College of General Practitioners* (1982), **32** 292–97)

Consultations and home visits	65%
Patient services (letters, telephone, repeat prescriptions etc.)	15%
Education and other health service work and administration	12%
Practice administration	8%
Total	100%

TRENDS

Intercontinental Medical Statistics data from 1969 to 1979 suggest certain trends in British general practice. Figure 9.4 is a summary.

Surgery consultations went up by 7%, home visits went down by 41% and other services such as repeat prescriptions, telephone, letters etc. went up by 250%. All face-to-face consultations decreased by 4.5%.

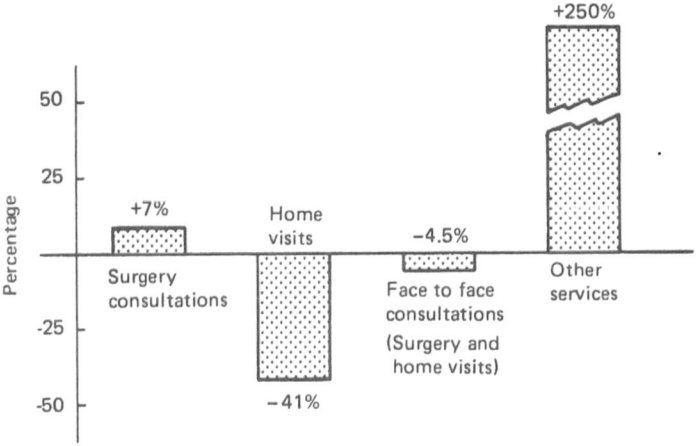

Figure 9.4   Trends in practice work load (1969–79), (from Intercontinental Medical Statistics Ltd)

47

WORK PROFILE OF GENERAL PRACTITIONERS IN A POPULATION OF 2500

Table 9.3 is an attempt to present the numbers involved as a composite model.

Table 9.3   Work profile per general practitioner

General practitioner work profile Population 2500	
Daily surgery consultations	30–40
Daily home visits	2–5
Other activities	? ? ?
Night visits	1 every 2 weeks

10
Prescribing by general practitioners

The cost of prescribing by general practitioners accounts for about 10% of the total costs of the NHS – and general practitioner prescribing makes up more than three-quarters of all prescribing costs within the NHS.

Now that the annual costs of the NHS are around £15 000 million a year, prescribing costs are about £1500 million or over £50 000 per general practitioner principal in the NHS (1982–83 rates).

PRESCRIPTION VOLUME AND COSTS PER PERSON

Table 10.1 and Figure 10.1 show the increases in annual volume and costs of prescribed drugs per person in the NHS from 1950 to 1980.

Table 10.1   NHS annual prescriptions per person and expenditure on NHS prescriptions per person at current and at 1949 prices

United Kingdom Year	NHS Prescriptions per person per year	Total expenditure per person on NHS prescriptions	
		Current prices	At 1949 prices
1950	4.80	£0.80	£0.78
1955	4.94	£1.11	£0.83
1960	4.68	£1.72	£1.12
1965	5.14	£2.67	£1.46
1970	5.52	£3.77	£1.66
1975	6.19	£8.01	£1.91
1980	6.68	£19.99	£2.43

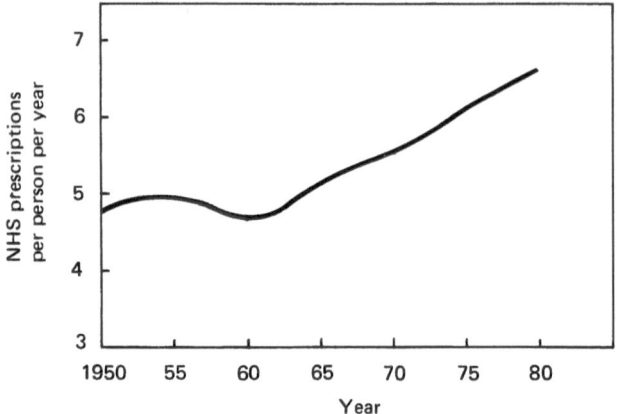

Figure 10.1   NHS annual prescriptions per person

In 1950 the mean number of prescriptions per person was 4.8, and by 1980 it had gone up to 6.68 – an increase in volume of almost 40%. The annual amount of money spent per person, at 1949 prices, went up 3-fold from 1950 to 1980.

It should be noted that the mean number of prescriptions per person now is almost seven, and that the mean number of annual general practitioner–patient consultations is 3.5. This suggests that about one-half of all prescriptions issued by GPs are for 'repeats' or for 'unseen consultations'.

Prescription charges currently (1982) are £1.30 per item on a prescription but it should be appreciated that in 1982 no fewer than 75% of all prescriptions issued were to persons exempt from such charges. In 1970 the exemption rate was 54%.

COSTS PER PRESCRIPTION

The total costs per prescription issued (Table 10.2 and Figure 10.2) at current prices (1982) are over £3 compared with 16.8 old pence in 1950 (at 1950 prices the 1980 rate would have been 37 pence).

Table 10.2   Annual mean total costs per NHS prescription

	Total costs per NHS prescription (pence)
1950	16.8
1955	22.5
1960	36.9
1965	52.0
1970	68.4
1975	129.3
1980	299.1 (37 pence at 1950 prices)

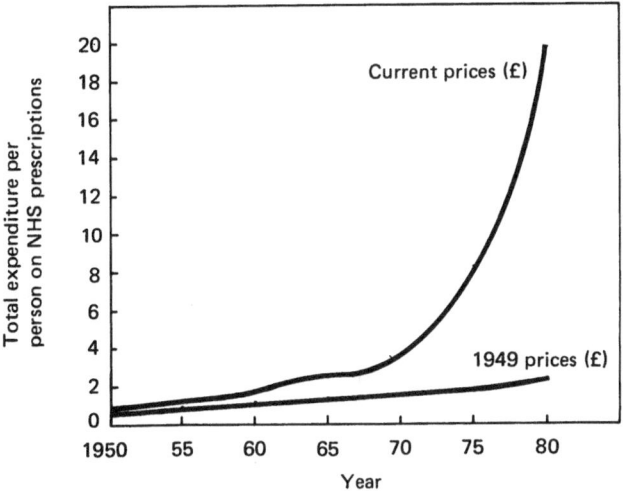

Figure 10.2   NHS annual expenditure per person at current and 1949 prices

PRESCRIPTIONS PER GENERAL PRACTITIONER – VOLUME AND COSTS

Table 10.3 shows the volume and costs of prescribing per general practitioner principal in the NHS.

It is of relevance and interest that over the past 15 years the annual total prescribing costs per general practitioner have been more than twice the annual net income per general practitioner.

51

Table 10.3   NHS prescriptions per general practitioner: annual volume and total costs

	Annual prescriptions per GP principal	Annual total costs of NHS prescriptions per GP principal
1950	10 955	£1864
1955	10 083	£2375
1960	9840	£3640
1965	11 625	£6042
1970	12 490	£8531
1975	13 308	£17 231
1980	13 123	£39 323
1982 (estimated)	13 000	£50 000

THERAPEUTIC GROUPS OF PRESCRIBED DRUGS

The proportions of various therapeutics groups prescribed and the average ingredient cost per prescription (Table 10.4) show

Table 10.4   Therapeutic groups of drugs: proportion of total and average net ingredient costs for 1979 (Great Britain)

Theraputic groups of drugs	Per cent of all prescriptions	Average net ingredient costs per prescription (pence)
Nervous system	24%	131
Gastrointestinal system	8%	206
Central venous system	15%	306
Respiratory system	10%	164
Rheumatic preparation	5%	417
Infections	12%	172
Haemopoiesis and blood preparations	3%	102
Skin	9%	130
Nutritional, Allergy Eye	7%	130
Others	5%	?
Dressings and appliances	2%	?
	100%	
(Total prescriptions 361 million)		(average = 196)

that drugs for the nervous system, cardiovascular system, infections (antibiotics) and respiratory conditions were the most frequently prescribed.

In terms of costs drugs for rheumatic conditions, dressings and appliances, cardiovascular system and hormones were the most expensive.

A better view of the more specific drugs prescribed can be obtained by looking at volume in millions of prescriptions in 1979 by general practitioners in Great Britain (Table 10.5).

Table 10.5

Nervous system	
hypnotics	18 million prescriptions
sedatives/tranquillizers	24 million prescriptions
anticonvulsants	4 million prescriptions
analgesics (major)	4 million prescriptions
analgesics (minor)	21 million prescriptions
antidepressants	8 million prescriptions
others	9 million prescriptions
Total (all)	88 million prescriptions
Gastrointestinal	
antacids	8 million prescriptions
antispasmodics	3 million prescriptions
gastrointestinal sedatives	3 million prescriptions
laxatives	5 million prescriptions
antidiarrhoeals	4 million prescriptions
others	3 million prescriptions
Total (all)	26 million prescriptions
Cardiovascular	
heart preparations	19 million prescriptions
diuretics	22 million prescriptions
antihypertensives	7 million prescriptions
vasodilators	3 million prescriptions
antimigraine agents	1 million prescriptions
others	3 million prescriptions
Total (all)	55 million prescriptions
Respiratory	
expectorants and cough suppressants	17 million prescriptions
asthma agents	14 million prescriptions
others	6 million prescriptions
Total (all)	37 million prescriptions

CONSUMPTION OF DRUGS – INTERNATIONAL DATA

Lest it be thought that we in Britain are high drug consumers, Figure 10.3 shows that we are actually in the lower ranges. Figure 10.3 also demonstrates the close relationship between the consumption of drugs and the national affluence; the more affluent the country the more drugs its people will consume.

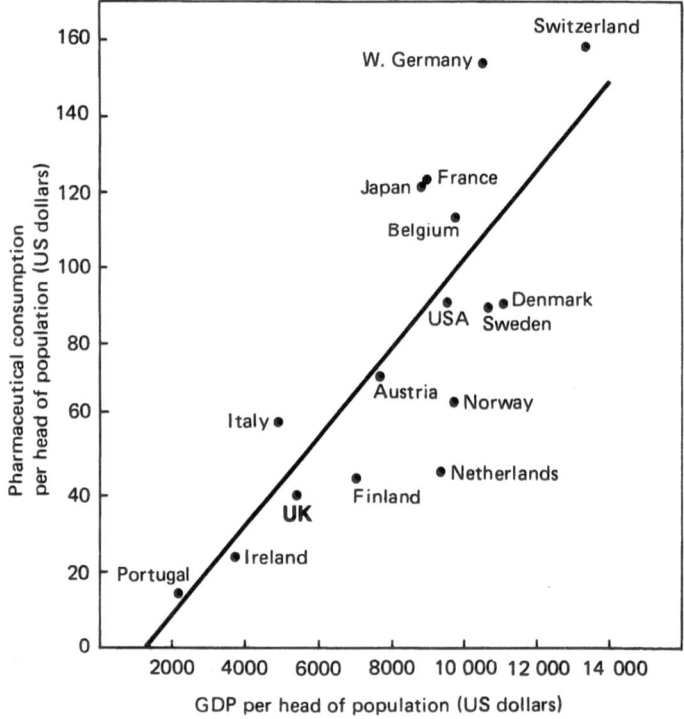

Figure 10.3 Relationships between drugs consumed per capita and gross domestic product in selected countries (from Office of Health Economics, 1982)

SOME IMPLICATIONS

* How many prescriptions are really necessary?
* Need they be so expensive?
* How can better prescribing be achieved?

11
General practitioners and the hospitals

General practice and the hospital service are essential complementary parts of the NHS. The pattern of cooperation is for general practitioners to refer their patients to hospital consultants at their outpatient clinics and to receive them back with reports or to admit emergencies direct to the wards. Accident and emergency departments usually accept patients without any need for prior referral.

Available data is crude and gross relating to average national rates. There are much more delicate differences of referral rates between individual practitioners.

USE OF HOSPITALS

Table 11.1 shows the utilization indices for NHS hospitals in England from 1949 to 1979 (Figures 11.1a-d).

Table 11.1   NHS hospitals (in England): indices of utilization in rates per 1000

	1949	1959	1969	1979
Hospital beds available	10.3	10.6	9.5	8.0
Inpatient admissions (deaths and discharges)	67	88	109	117
New referrals to out-patient departments	140	159	166	167
Accident and emergency (new cases)	89	121	166	198

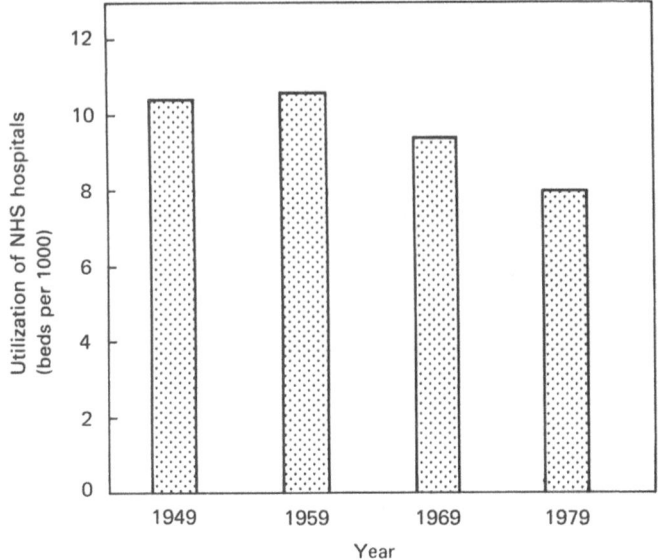

Figure 11.1a

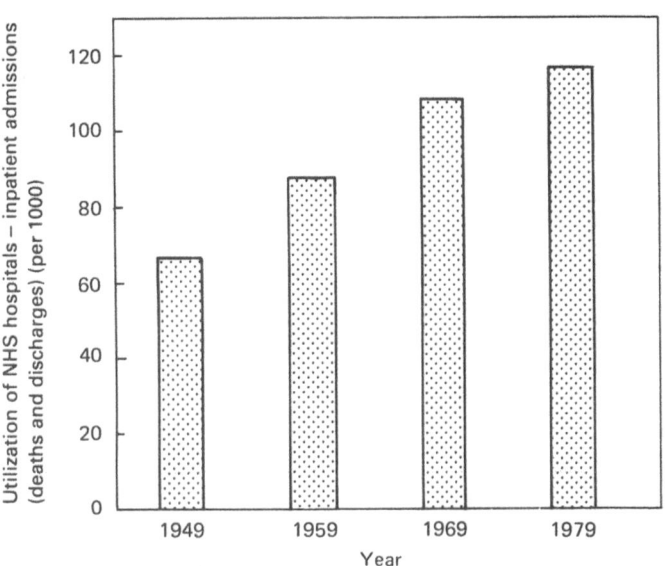

Figure 11.1b

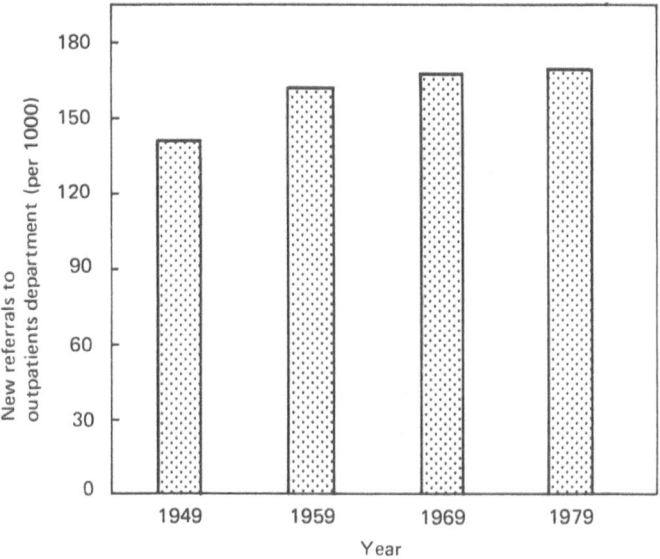

Figure 11.1c

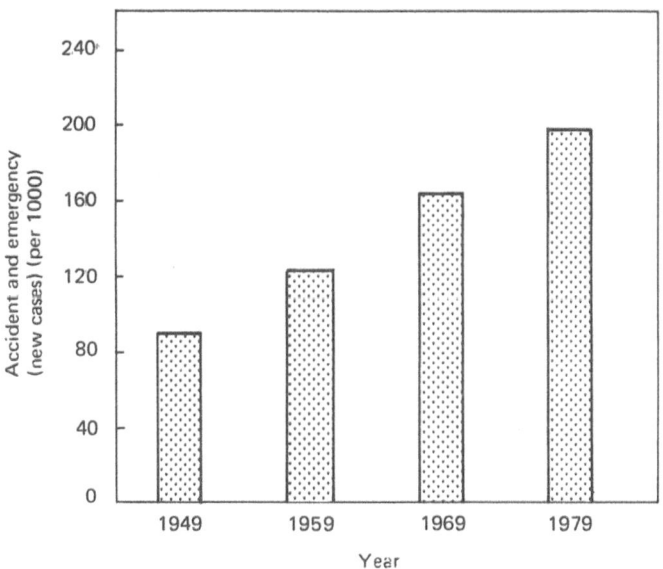

Figure 11.1d

57

Available numbers of hospital beds were reduced but the rates admitted (discharges and deaths) have increased steadily. New referrals to outpatient departments increased from 1949 to 1969 and have levelled off since, and the use of accident and emergency departments has more than doubled.

It should be appreciated that in a year a large proportion of our population will use our hospital services (Table 11.2 and Figure 11.2).

Table 11.2   Proportion of total population using hospital services

Admitted to hospital	12%
New referrals to outpatient departments	17%
New attendances to accident and emergency departments	20%
Total attending hospital	? 35–40%
Consultation with general practitioner	65%

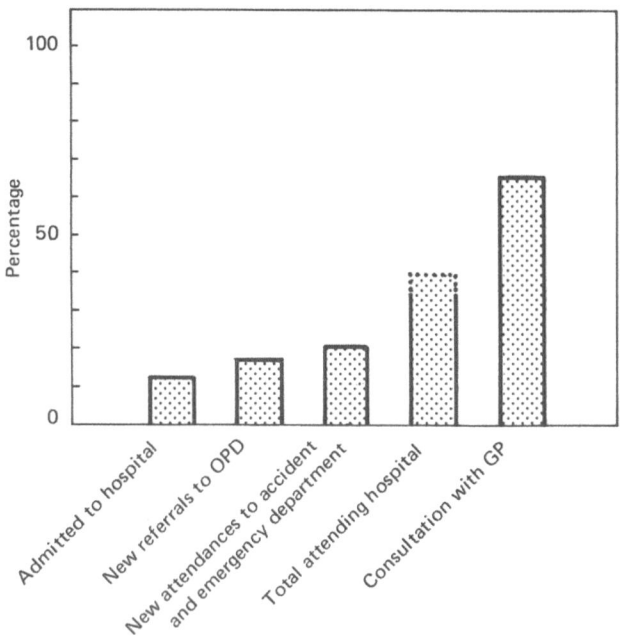

Figure 11.2   Proportion of total population using hospital services

We do not know what percentage of the whole population will use NHS hospital services in any year because the same persons may use all three parts of the service. In theory it may be that almost one-half may be seen at hospital – but it is more likely to be much less, say 35–40%. Note that about 65% of the population will consult their general practitioner at least once a year.

NUMBERS OF REFERRALS PER GENERAL PRACTITIONER

A convenient way of viewing hospital referrals is to relate them to an average hypothetical practice of 2500 persons. Tables 11.3-4 and Figures 11.3-4 show such numbers for hospital admissions and for new referrals to outpatient departments.

Table 11.3   Annual hospital admissions per 2500

Specialty	Numbers
Surgical	
general surgery	54
gynaecology	26
trauma–orthopaedics	25
ear, nose and throat	15
others	20
	140
Medical	
general medical	40
paediatrics	12
psychiatry	11
geriatrics	10
others	7
	80
Obstetrics	30
Others	25
Total	275

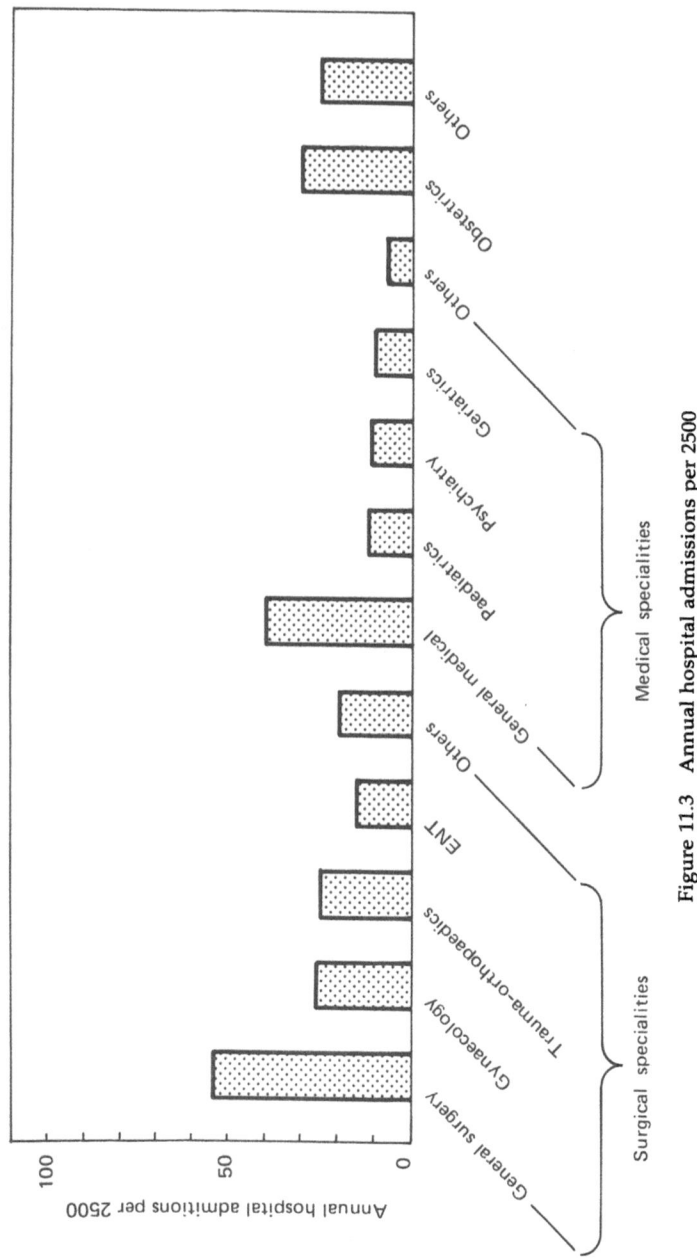

Figure 11.3 Annual hospital admissions per 2500

Table 11.4   Annual new referrals to outpatient departments per 2500

Specialty	Numbers
Surgical	
general surgical	50
gynaecological	30
trauma–orthopaedics	60
ear, nose and throat	30
ophthalmology	30
others	50
	250
Medical	
general medical	25
paediatrics	10
psychiatry	12
dermatology	25
chest	15
others	23
	110
Obstetrics	30
Others	25
Total	415

DOMICILIARY CONSULTATIONS

A unique service of the NHS is the domiciliary consultation. It was introduced into the NHS from its very beginning (1948) to perpetuate and encourage the valuable bedside consultation between specialist and general practitioner in the patient's home. The specialist receives a fee for such a service, the general practitioner does not.

Unfortunately with time the 'consultation' has tended to become more of a 'visit' by the specialist alone to the home, without the general practitioner. It is likely that a domiciliary bedside consultation occurs at less than one-half of such visits.

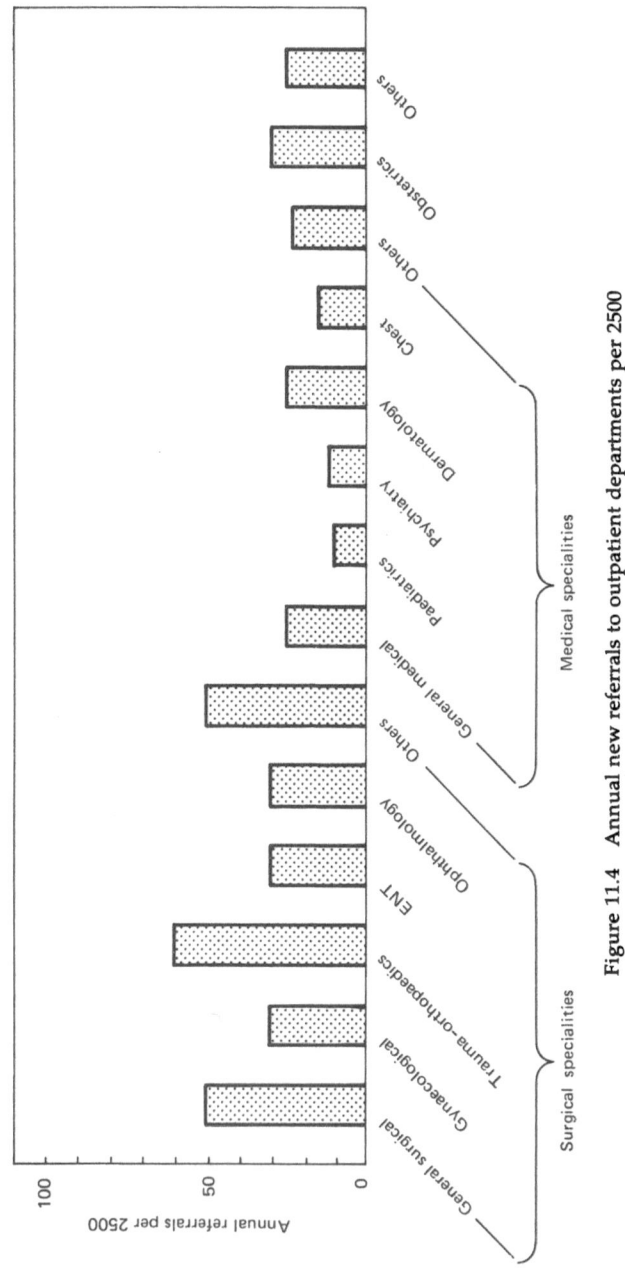

Figure 11.4 Annual new referrals to outpatient departments per 2500

The average annual numbers of domiciliary visits (consultations) for each specialist in various specialties is shown in Table 11.5 and Figure 11.5. The average number of domiciliary visits per NHS specialist in 1979–80 was 37.3, that is one every 10 days.

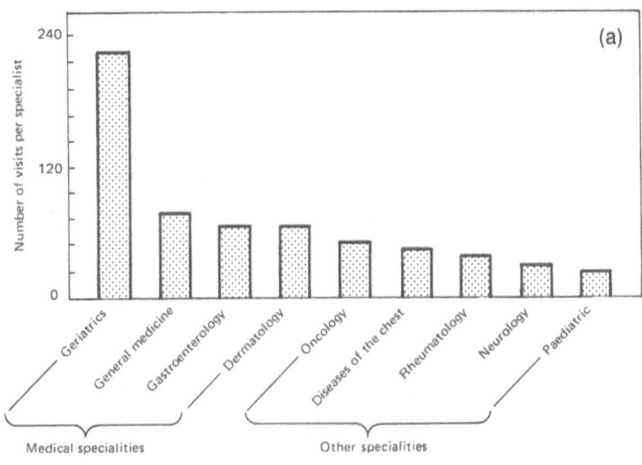

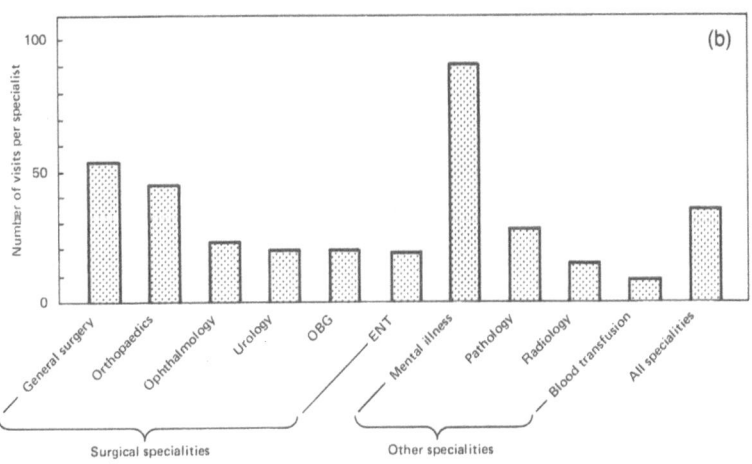

Figure 11.5a, b   NHS domiciliary visits: average annual numbers per specialist in various specialties (1978-9)

Table 11.5   NHS domiciliary visits: average annual numbers per specialist in various specialties (1978–9)

Specialty	Average annual number of domiciliary visits per specialist
Medical	
geriatrics	217
general medicine	78
gastroenterology	63
dermatology	63
Medical	
oncology	54
diseases of the chest	51
rheumatology	49
neurology	35
paediatric	25
Surgical	
general surgery	54
orthopaedics	45
ophthalmology	23
urology	20
obstetrics and gynaecology	20
ear, nose and throat	19
Mental illness	91
Pathology	28
Radiology	15
Blood transfusion	9
All specialties	37

12
The general practitioner in the hospital

One of the bad effects of the NHS has been the separation of general practice and hospital services. It is unusual, except in the few general practitioner hospitals, for general practitioners to admit and take responsible care of their own patients in local hospitals. A different state of affairs exists in the United States and Canada where primary physicians have access to hospital beds.

It is likely that the quality of general practice and the satisfaction both of patients and doctors are greater where it is customary for general practitioners to have access to hospital beds to admit and care for their own patients.

In spite of the sad lack of general practitioner community hospitals, paradoxically about one-quarter to one-third of general practitioners have some formal links with local hospitals through their work as clinical assistants working in specialist units – usually in outpatient departments – but not with their own patients.

GENERAL PRACTITIONERS IN HOSPITALS

It is estimated that there are about 6000 general practitioner clinical assistants in the NHS, or just under one-quarter. There are also those who have other local associations.

Most of these clinical assistants are in the specialties of general medicine, geriatrics, accident and emergency, psychiatry, obstetrics and gynaecology, anaesthetics and paediatrics.

They have no career structure or security of tenure – but in the newer appointment of hospital practitioner there is progressive increase in pay and security of tenure. By 1981 there were 864 hospital practitioners in England and Wales.

GENERAL PRACTITIONER COMMUNITY HOSPITALS

There are 423 NHS general practitioner hospitals – 350 in England and Wales, 62 in Scotland and eleven in Northern Ireland. They provide care for about 18% of our population (10 million), and 4000 general practitioners (16% of all general practitioners) work in them, spending 10% of their working time there.

GENERAL PRACTITIONER OBSTETRIC UNITS

There are about 150 NHS general practitioner obstetric units/ hospitals. Only one-quarter of general practitioner community hospitals have an attached obstetric unit.

The trends are to close down small isolated obstetric units and to replace them by general practitioner units in district general hospitals.

13
Costs of health care

The cost of health care is soaring all over the world, and inflation alone is not responsible. Taking account of inflation the cost of the NHS has increased 3-fold in real terms since its inception.

There are few data on quality – only a collection of indices and rough figures.

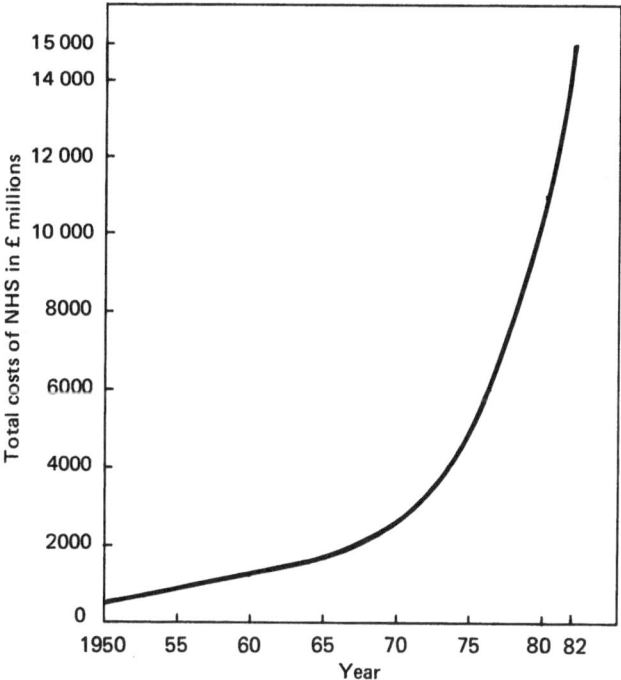

Figure 13.1   Total costs of NHS 1949–80 (not adjusted for inflation)

TOTAL NHS EXPENDITURE

Health expenditure costs may be measured and presented in various ways. Each has its own messages.

* *Crude costs.* Accounting and presenting the total costs each year is simple, but limited in value because of inflation. Figure 13.1 shows that the increase in costs of the NHS between 1949 (when it was £437 million) and 1980 (£11 875 million) has been of the order of 2600% (1982 costs will have been £15 000 million).

* *Costs adjusted for inflation.* As a fairer estimate of the real increase in costs of the NHS, Figure 13.2 shows the total NHS costs at 1949 prices and adjusted for inflation. Here, the increase between 1949 and 1980 is about 320% (from £437 million to £1450 million).

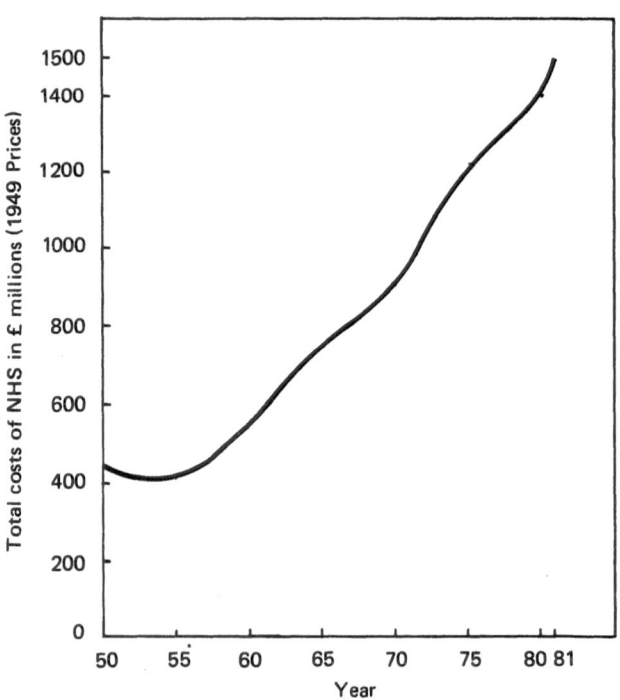

Figure 13.2   Total costs of NHS 1949–80 (at 1949 prices and adjusted for inflation)

* *Costs per head of population.* There is a fond illusion that the NHS is 'free'. The best way to dispel this myth is to show how much the NHS costs per head of the population – that is, every man, woman and child. In 1980 the estimated cost of paying for our NHS was no less than £200 per person per year. In other words, an average family of father, mother and two children will be paying out of taxation and direct payments £800 per year, or £16 per week. This has gone up from £9 per person per year in 1949 (an increase of 220%) (Figure 13.3).

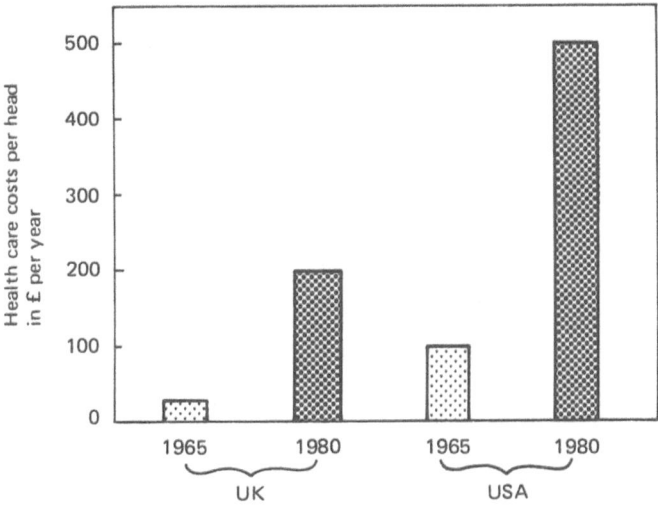

Figure 13.3   Health care costs per head in the United Kingdom and the United States, 1969–79

To show that the increases are not purely a British phenomenon, comparative rates for the United States and the United Kingdom from 1965 to 1979 are given. The apparent increases have been more than twice as high in the United Kingdom (eight times) than in the United States (five times), but our inflation rate has been twice as high also. The rates of increase in costs per head have therefore been similar. However, note that the total annual health care costs for a family of four in the United States in 1980 were £2000, or £40 per week.

* *NHS costs as a percentage of the gross national product (GNP).*
Another way of assessing health care costs is to relate these
costs to the gross national product (i.e. what the country
earns and is worth). Figure 13.4 shows that the amount of
the gross national product spent on the NHS from 1965 to
1980. From 1949 to 1980 it increased by about 50% (from 3.92
to 5.70% of the gross national product).

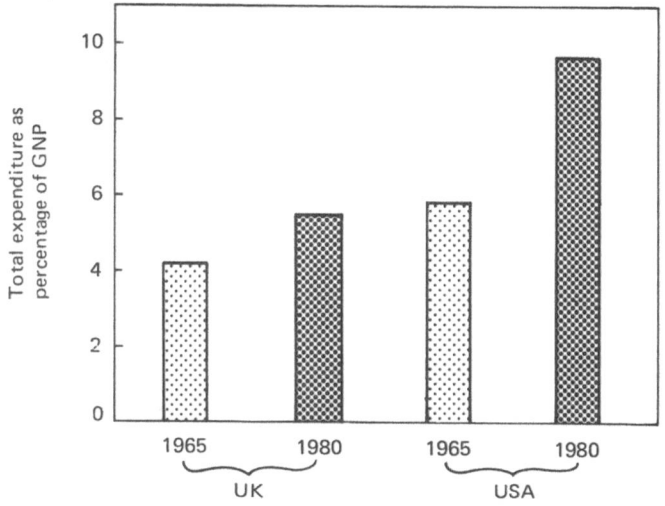

Figure 13.4   Total NHS expenditure as a percentage of the gross national
product 1949–80

COMPARISONS WITH OTHER SYSTEMS

How does our spending compare with other countries? Figures
13.5 and 13.6 show that we are low spenders, but not as low as
Japan.

Figure 13.5 demonstrates that the per capita expenditure is
related directly to the gross national product per capita, and
Figure 13.6 shows that the higher the national income (expressed
as gross national product per capita) the greater the percentage
of gross national product that will be spent on health care.
Therefore, if we improve our gross national product then we can
expect more money to be devoted to the NHS.

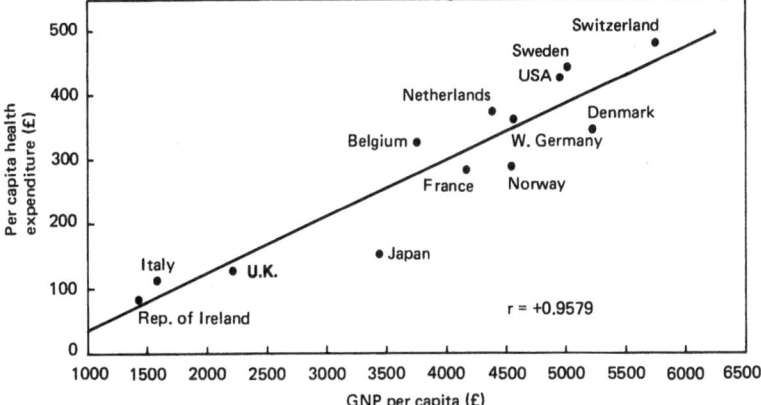

Figure 13.5   Regression of per capita health expenditure on the gross national product (Office of Health Economics, 1979)

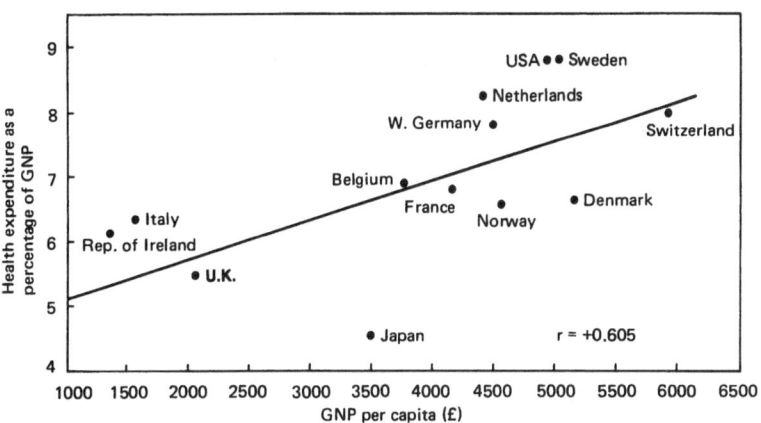

Figure 13.6   Regression of health service expenditure as a percentage of the gross national product on gross national product per capita (Office of Health Economics, 1979)

WHAT DO WE SPEND THE MONEY ON?

The proportion of NHS expenditure on various services is shown in Figure 13.7. Since 1950 the proportion of hospital expenditure has increased from 55% to 63% (1974), and that for general practice has decreased from 10% (1950) to 6% (1974).

71

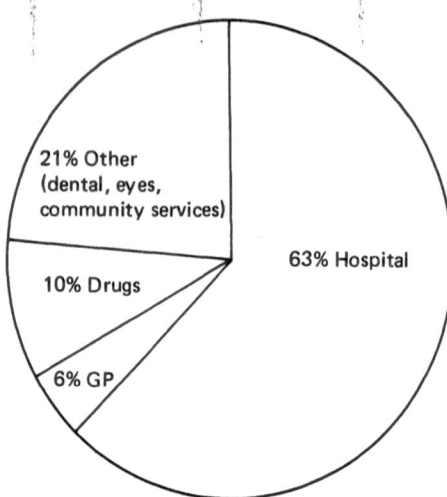

Figure 13.7   NHS expenditure: proportion spent on each service

WHERE DOES THE MONEY COME FROM?

Figure 13.8 shows that most of the money for the NHS comes from central government taxation (88%).

The proportion from direct insurance contribution is only 10% and patient payment for drugs, dental, opthalmic and other services contributes but 2%.

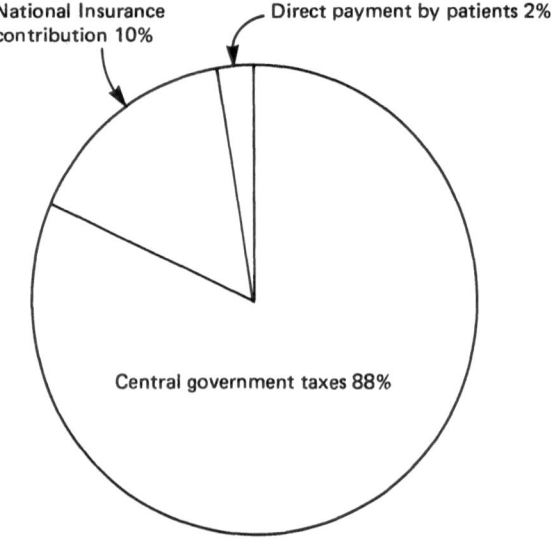

Figure 13.8   Sources of finance in the NHS

14
The Royal College of General Practitioners

The College was founded in 1952 as an act of faith and confidence in the aftermath of the Second World War by general practitioners who believed that they worked in a special branch of health care with its own skills, expertise, methods and tools. They believed that for general practice to flourish, improve and prosper demanded special education, training and research.

The history of the first 25 years of the College has been written (RCGP, 1983) and it records the early problems and difficulties that had to be overcome before its goals were achieved.

NUMBERS
The College is composed of fellows, members and associates – the 10 000th was reached in 1982. One third of all GP's are now members or associates of the College.

In 1981 there were:

Honorary fellows	37
Fellows	892
Members	6917
Associates	1848
Total	9694

The growth over the years is shown in Figure 14.1.

MEMBERSHIP BY EXAMINATION
Since 1965 membership of the RCGP has been by examination, and Figure 14.1 shows that the proportions of fellows and

members who have entered in this way has increased and is now well over one-half.

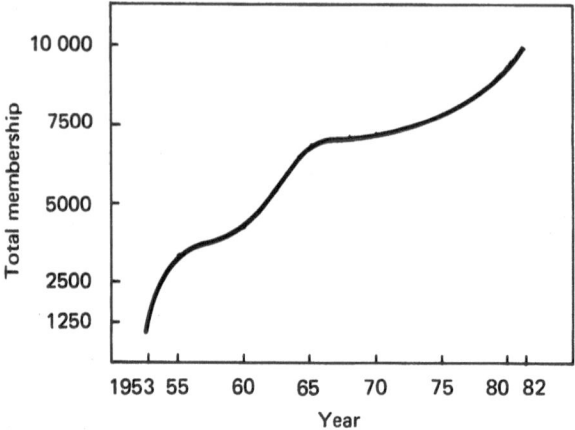

Figure 14.1   Total membership of the Royal College of General Practitioners

THE MRGCP EXAMINATION

Over a thousand candidates take the MRGCP each year now and the figures for 1979–80 in Table 14.1 show an overall pass rate of 60%.

Table 14.1   MRGCP Examination 1979–80: candidates and pass rates

	Per cent candidates	Per cent pass rate
NHS: GP principal	42	52
Assistant	4	38
Trainee	46	70
Hospital doctor	3	58
Services (HM Forces)	3	66
Others	2	38
(Foreign medical graduates)	(12)	(6)
All groups	100% (1046 candidates, males 82% females 18%)	60%

The highest pass rates for the various groups of candidates are in the trainee and in candidates from H.M. Forces (Services) categories.

AGE OF COLLEGE MEMBERS

The age grouping of the College membership (Table 14.2) compared with that of all NHS general practitioners shows that there are more very young members in the College and more older members too. This is explained by new members coming from trainees; the older members are the original foundation supporters. It does confirm the relatively low support given to the college by those NHS general practitioners now in the 40-49 age group.

Table 14.2   RCGP members and NHS general practitioners: percentages in age groups

Age	under 30	30+	40+	50+	60+	70+	
RCGP members	6	32	16	25	15	6	100
NHS general practitioners	2	30	30	25	10	3	100

15
Future needs

GENERAL TRENDS

General practice, or primary health care, the oldest branch of medicine, has been steadily transformed in the past 10–15 years. It has shed the image of being an outmoded, outdated and less than necessary cottage industry in the modern medical world filled with the bright new technologies of hospital-based specialties. It has created for itself a new vitality with new roles and new goals and acceptance and recognition that it is an essential level of care in all health care systems.

General practice has progressed from a soft option for the less successful and less ambitious medical graduate to the first-career choice of the brightest medical students.

On the wider stage the World Health Organization is basing its hopes for 'Health for All – 2000 AD' on a strong well-developed and strongly supported level of primary health care.

Everywhere there have been attempts to promote primary health care, but in the United Kingdom we have had the benefits of long-established traditions of 'good general practice'. These were firmly reinforced in 1948 by giving general practice its own independent administration and organization within the National Health Service.

Since 1948, slowly at first but rapidly in the past decade, general practice has defined its own content and problems, its own roles, its own methods and techniques, its own education and training and its own research. This has not been solely a British experience, it has been happening simultaneously in many countries.

Notable among the general trends in British general practice have been:

* a tighter modern system of organization and administration;
* teamwork between general practitioners and other members of the primary health care team;
* a movement away from solo single-handed practice towards groups working from health centres and group premises;
* rethinking the objectives of care and promotion of prevention and better self-care through health education, earlier diagnosis and long-term supervision.

SPECIFIC NEEDS

In spite of the changes there have been no movements towards very large groups and partnerships. Overall the average size of a practice is still between three and four general practitioners. Each such group will provide care for about 10 000 persons.

A major future need is to produce and implement a reasonable plan for improving the health of such a population, including preventive measures, health promotion and maintenance and creating practice policies for managing common disorders, chronic diseases, acute major situations and social problems, not only in individual patients but in the community as a whole.

No longer is it enough to provide available and accessible primary care for those who seek it. The challenges must be faced of seeking out early subclinical disorders and potentially dangerous personal habits and attempting to correct them.

Clinical disorders and problems must continue as a top priority. Patients seek cure, relief and comfort for their physical illnesses and discomforts.

The common and less common disorders of general practice have not been subjected to intensive research and study. Unless we know much more about the nature, course and outcome of such common bread-and-butter diseases then general practitioners cannot manage them effectively, efficiently and economically.

Although clinical matters are of prime importance *behavioural, emotional and social problems* must also be recognized as important. They must be researched further to discover how they may be recognized, understood by patients as well as doctors, and what useful measures can be taken to help those affected.

The *primary health care team and 'teamwork'* have become popular expressions suggesting hopeful collaborative endeavours and results.

A practice group of four general practitioners may include another 10 to 15 members of the team – secretaries-receptionists, nurses, health visitors, midwives and others.

The rapid evolution of the primary health care team has scarcely produced experiments to test the many possible ways in which the various members of the team may function. All now are trained and skilled and the non-medical members could undertake more tasks and roles previously reserved for doctors.

Another future need is to encourage experiments and trials to test new roles and tasks for the primary health care team. We need to know more about who does what best in general practice.

The most expensive part of any health system is the remuneration of doctors, nurses and others involved in providing care. It is amazing, therefore, that there are no reliable ways in which *national medical manpower policies* can be devised. We do not know how many general practitioners are *really* necessary – nor the right numbers of hospital doctors, nurses, administrative staff and other personnel; these have been increasing in the NHS every year since it began..

As a corollary to any experiments into the roles of the primary health care team it is necessary to try and decide how many doctors, nurses and medical secretaries we really need.

General practitioners tend to work alone and in relative isolation – even though they may be members of a group practice. Each one of us tends to develop his or her own *particular habits of work, prescribing and hospital referrals.*

Future needs should examine our patterns of work, prescribing and hospital referrals and compare them with those of our colleagues – not for any critical or derogatory reasons, but in attempts to discover how we carry out our tasks and how we may do them better.

NEEDS FOR THE FUTURE

The present state of general practice in the NHS is that we seem to have the resources to do the job but that we are uncertain on what our roles should be and how best to try and achieve them.

To promote better care that is more effective, efficient and economic more research studies, experiments and trials are needed to provide useful and reliable information and facts on which we might be able to take decisions on our future.

* We must have data on how best to manage the specific common diseases, disorders and problems of general practice. It is of little value to rely on results from hospital practice, where diseases, problems and situations are different.

* The computer and its allied technology provide challenges and opportunities for general practice.

* We must try and produce protocols for 'good general practice' for our own practices in which policies are spelt out for prevention, health promotion, management and review of results.

* New roles and tasks for the primary health care team should be tested and evaluated. It is likely that general practitioners underestimate the potential of nurses, health visitors and medical secretaries in undertaking new tasks.

* Probably the most important future need is to inculcate the spirit of self-enquiry and self-checking to examine and analyse our own work in our practices in order to define weaknesses and seek improvements.

Index

Journal of
The Royal College
of General Practitioners
The British Journal of General Practice

The *Journal of the Royal College of General Practitioners* was one of the first academic journals of general practice in the world. It is published monthly and contains editorials, original articles, a news section, book reviews, and correspondence covering all aspects of modern general practice. Its policy is to describe and comment on all new developments in general practice and it publishes exclusively many of the important policy decisions and reports of the Royal College of General Practitioners.

The *Journal* is sent to all Fellows, Honorary Fellows, Members, Associates and corresponding Associates of the Royal College of General Practitioners, and also to a growing number of private subscribers including university postgraduate medical centres, hospital libraries, institutions, and individuals in over 40 different countries of the world.

All subscribers receive the *Reports from General Practice* and *Journal Supplements* free of charge with the *Journal* when these are published. The *Occasional Papers* are not distributed free but are available whilst in print from the address below at prices shown regularly in the *Journal* and other College publications. The *Reports from General Practice, Journal Supplements* and *Occasional Papers* cover in depth aspects of special importance to general practice and form some of the most authoritative data and source documents available.

The annual subscription to the *Journal* is £40.00 (£45.00 or $100.00 overseas) post free. Single copies are £3.50 (£4.00 or $8.50 overseas). Orders and payments should be sent to the Publication Sales Department, Royal College of General Practitioners, 14 Princes Gate, Hyde Park, London SW7 1PU.

Vocational trainees can apply to the Membership Secretary of the College for Associate membership at the specially reduced rate of £20.00, which includes receipt of the *Journal, Supplements* and *Reports from General Practice* when published.

The following publications from the Royal College of General Practitioners can be obtained from the Publications Sales Department of the Royal College of General Practitioners, 14 Princes Gate, Hyde Park, London SW7 1PU. All prices include postage and payment should be made with order.

REPORTS FROM GENERAL PRACTICE
18. Health and Prevention in Primary Care £3.00
19. Prevention of Arterial Disease in General Practice ... £3.00
20. Prevention of Psychiatric Disorders in General Practice £3.00
21. Family Planning – An Exercise in Preventive Medicine £2.25
22. Healthier Children – Thinking Prevention £5.50

OCCASIONAL PAPERS
4. A System of Training for General Practice (2nd edn) ... £3.00
6. Some Aims for Training for General Practice £2.75
7. Doctors on the Move £3.00
8. Patients and their Doctors 1977 ... ... £3.00
9. General Practitioners and Postgraduate Education in the Northern Region £3.00
10. Selected Papers from the Eighth World Conference on Family Medicine £3.75
11. Section 63 Activities £3.75
12. Hypertension in Primary Care £3.75
13. Computers in Primary Care £3.00
14. Education for Co-operation in Health and Social Work £3.00
15. The Measurement of the Quality of General Practitioner Care £3.00
16. A Survey of Primary Care in London £4.00
17. Patient Participation in General Practice £3.75
18. Fourth National Trainee Conference £3.75
19. Inner Cities £3.00
20. Medical Audit in General Practice £3.25
21. The Influence of Trainers on Trainees in General Practice £3.25

BOOKS
The Future General Practitioner £7.50*
Trends in General Practice 1979 ... ... £5.00*
Computers and the General Practitioner £10.50
Epidemiology and Research in a General Practice £10.50
A History of the Royal College of General Practitioners £12.00†
Members' Reference Book £17.50
Present State and Future Needs in General Practice ... £5.50

*£1.00 less for members of the College †£2.00 less for members of the College